A NEW VIEW OF HEALTHY EATING

SIMPLE INTUITIVE COOKING WITH REAL WHOLE FOODS

MELANIE A. ALBERT

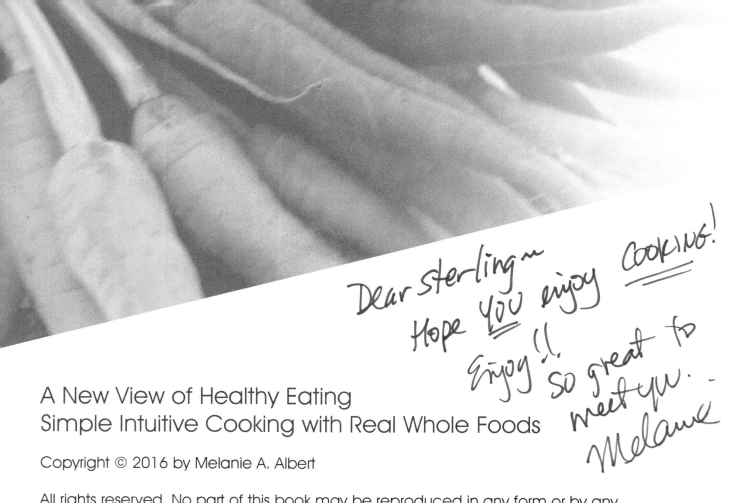

Dear Sterling~
Hope YOU enjoy COOKING!
Enjoy!!. So great to
meet you. -
Melanie

A New View of Healthy Eating
Simple Intuitive Cooking with Real Whole Foods

The content of this book is for general instruction only. Each person's physical, emotional, and spiritual condition is unique. The instruction in this book is not intended to replace or interrupt the reader's relationship with a physician or other professional. Please consult your doctor for matters pertaining to your specific health and diet.

To learn more about "A New View of Healthy Eating. Simple Intuitive Cooking with Real Whole Foods" visit www.NewViewHealthyEating.com

To contact the publisher and author, visit www.EXPNutrition.com

ISBN: 978-0-9862888-2-1

Library of Congress Control Number: 2016951185

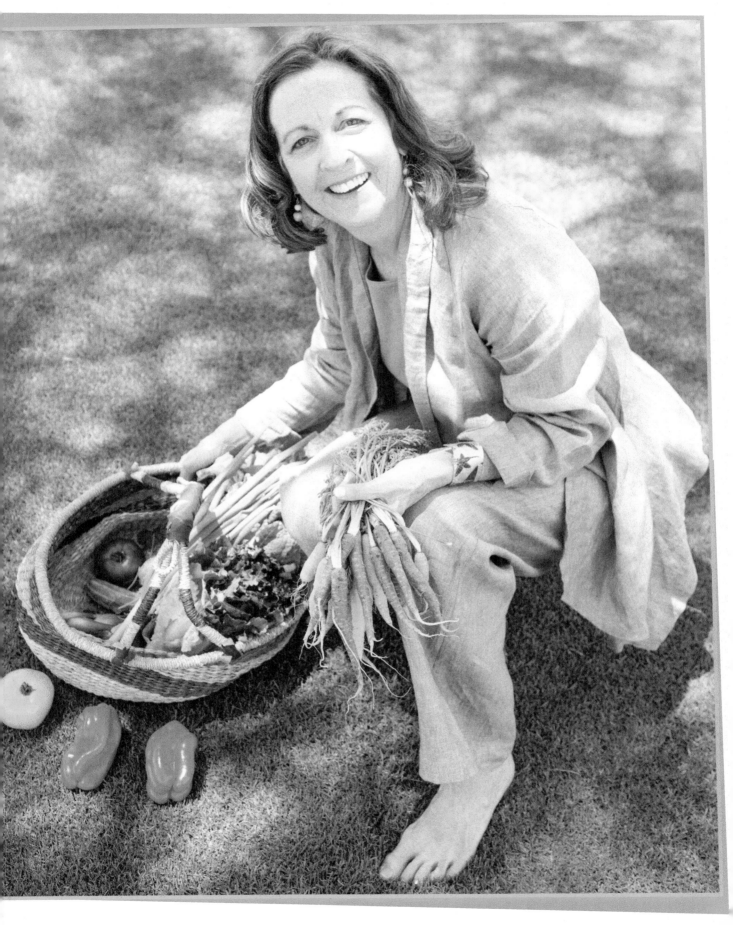

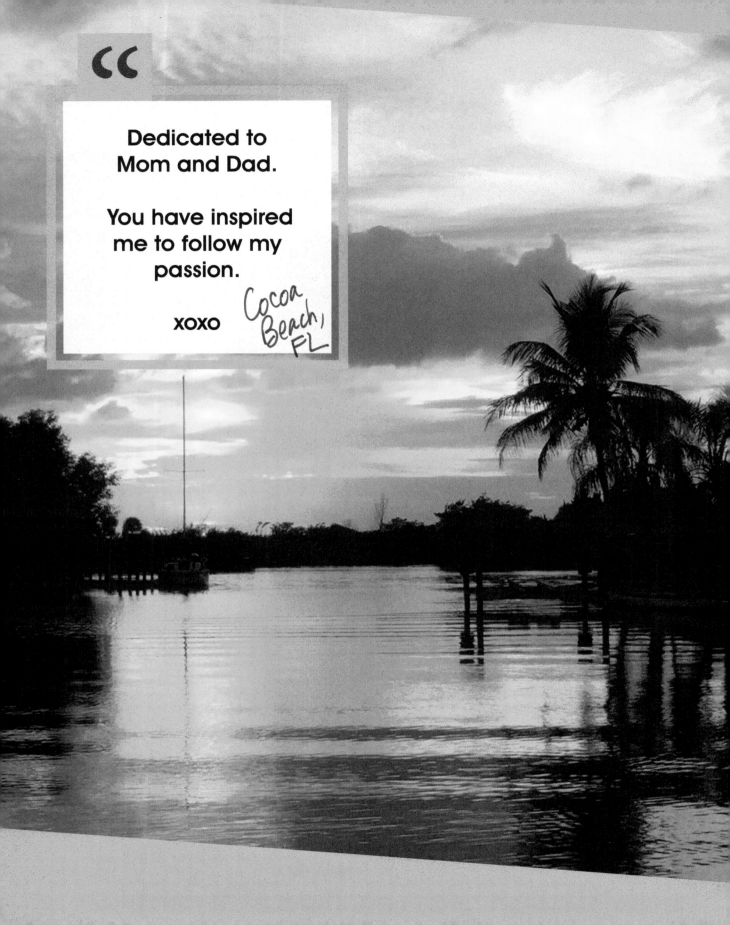

"

Dedicated to
Mom and Dad.

You have inspired
me to follow my
passion.

xoxo   Cocoa
Beach,
FL

THANK YOU

Dr. Andrew Weil, Integrative Medicine Pioneer
Thank you for the honor to work with you and your organization for nearly a decade.

Joshua Rosenthal, Founder Institute for Integrative Nutrition
Thank you for the foundation education to take my passions and skills to the world.

KC Miller, Founder Southwest Institute of Healing Arts
Thank you for the opportunity to teach and inspire students about intuitive whole foods cooking.

Former NFL Players and Families
Thank you for trusting me to come into your homes to guide you to cook with real whole foods.
Seth Joyner, Dave Krieg, John Bronson
Jerome and Tanya Daniels
NFL wife, Ericka Lassiter

Megan Holland, Director at Hall of Fame Players Classic and Foundation
Thank you for always inviting me to be part of NFL Hall of Fame Super Bowl activities to inspire the players.

Diana Gregory, Founder Gregory's Fresh Market
Thank you for the opportunities to guide seniors in Arizona to prepare simple, good-for-us food.

The First Tee of Phoenix
Thank you for the golf events to inspire the sports youth to have fun with food.

My Students and Friends
Thank you for all the support with your generous compliments and encouragement while teaching and writing.

My Brothers and Your Families
Thank you for always supporting me through the years with my 'crazy' food ideas, experimenting with my nieces and nephews, and photos – way before food photos were popular.

I appreciate each and every one of you.

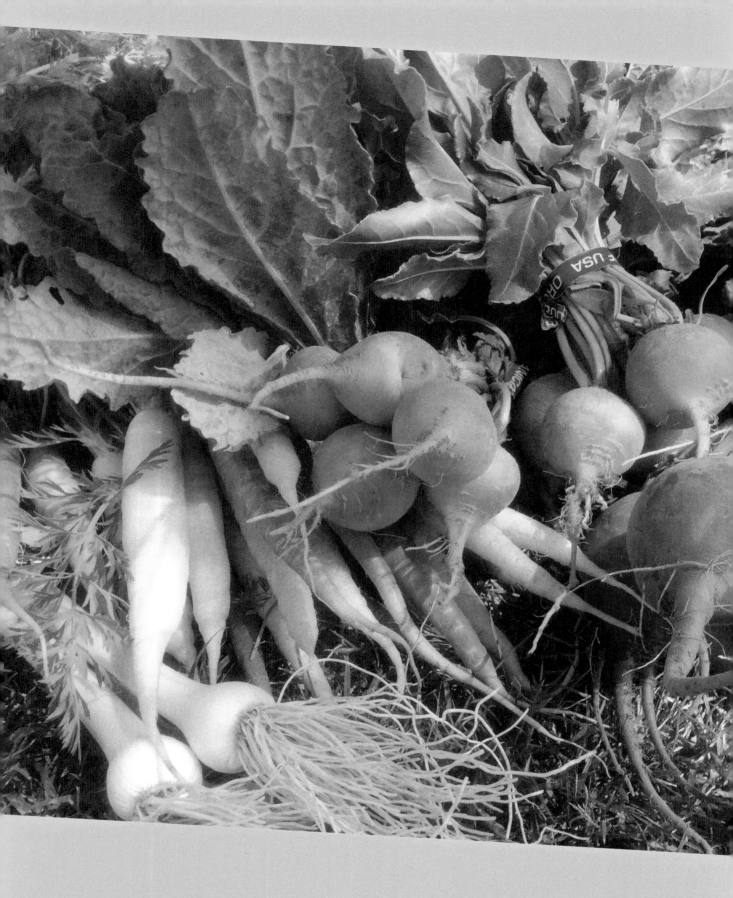

TABLE OF CONTENTS

INTRODUCTION

I initially learned first-hand the power of eating real whole foods over 20 years ago, in 1993, when my Mom, then 65 years old, was diagnosed with stage IV breast cancer and the conventional doctors gave her six months to live. Mom had the mastectomy, chemo, and radiation, and I left my successful corporate marketing career to be with her and my dad. I read nutrition books (there were only a few at the time). I had already stopped eating meat in the early 1980's when I noticed that my body could not metabolize it and I intuitively started eating organic food in the early 1990's. After Mom's cancer diagnosis, I developed a plant-based way of eating for my parents, and with Mom's positive outlook on life, I'm happy to say that as I write this, my mom is now 86 years old and very happy living in Cocoa Beach, Florida with my dad.

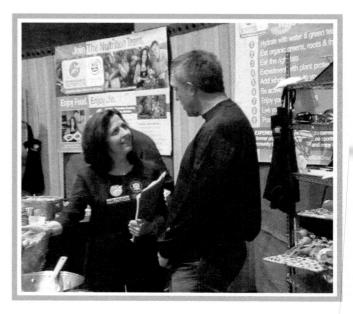

From 2008 to 2011, during four Super Bowl weeks, I was honored to have been active in numerous events with former NFL and Hall of Fame players by offering Super Bowl branded healthy lifestyle products, nutrition education and healthy organic catering.

In 2009, while talking with former NFL players during Super Bowl XLIII week in Tampa, I learned about the serious health issues – obesity, diabetes, heart disease, and pain – experienced by retired NFL players of the 1970's. I intuitively knew that these health issues could be positively improved through food. For several years, I went into the kitchens of a number of former NFL players and their wives and taught them simple ways to cook healthy meals with whole foods. In 2011 my company, Experience Nutrition, was honored to be an official Health and Wellness Partner of the NFL Alumni Association.

During the last few years, my teaching about sound nutrition through hands-on, interactive, intuitive cooking classes, workshops, demos, and retreats with real whole foods has expanded. I'm honored to teach Whole Foods Cooking and Conscious Eating courses at the private college Southwest Institute of Healing Arts and I have led intuitive eating sessions at the Spirit of Yoga in Tempe, Arizona.

I'm grateful to present healthy eating and whole food cooking education during employee meetings, conferences, events, and retreats with organizations such as the City of Phoenix, Food Day Phoenix, Marquette General Hospital Nutrition and Medicine Conference, Parkinson's Wellness Recovery, The Mankind Project, Gregory's Fresh Market, Whole Foods Market, and Yoga Rocks the Park. I also love inspiring our youth to get excited about eating healthy food with organizations such as Desert Vista High School, The First Tee of Phoenix, Future for Kids, Phoenix Suns/Mercury Kids Camps, and Arizona Youth Sports Day.

I've learned first-hand with thousands of people the value of simple cooking with a few basic culinary techniques using easy-to-prepare recipes, and then intuitively creating beautiful, tasty meals with local, in-season, real whole foods.

I realized that the hands-on interactive nutrition and intuitive cooking programs that I had created and been teaching were so powerful and had positively changed the lives of so many people who took part in my classes, workshops, speaking engagements, retreats, and demos that I wanted to reach more people. As a result, I decided to write this book and create a handy

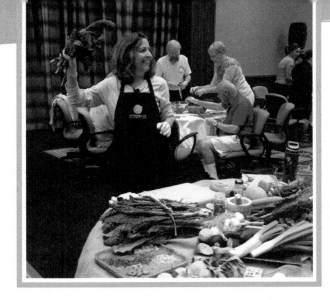

This book is a result of my experiences in the kitchens of former NFL players and their families, with cooking classes and workshops for holistic practitioners and yoga students, and with cooking demos for organizations. You'll learn simple culinary techniques and methods (e.g., cooking with a bamboo steamer; shopping for the right knife for you) and nutrition tips (e.g., protein-rich plant foods). You'll also learn how to intuitively cook plant-based dishes (and wild salmon) to create simple, delicious meals for yourself, your family, and your friends.

companion motivational healthy eating card deck, as well as shoot videos and create online programs to encourage health, nutrition, and fun in the kitchen. My goal through these efforts is to inspire and motivate more people by working with organizations, non-profits, retreats, and holistic practitioners.

So that you get the most out of this book, I recommend that you begin with the first three sections. The first section outlines my philosophies about food. The second will guide you through the process of getting your kitchen ready for healthy eating success, as it offers information about shopping for organic real whole foods. The third section will prepare you with the essential kitchen tools and foods for whole food cooking success.

It's important to mention that I am not a professional chef, but I've learned how to cook with basic culinary techniques. I have taught and inspired others to do the same. I've extended my culinary expertise with cooking training in the Plant-Based Professional Certification with the Rouxbe Cooking School.

After that, the book is organized by types of food and includes simple recipes, culinary cooking techniques, and nutrition tips. Chapters are organized into nine delicious whole food categories: Raw Veggies; Soups, Salads, and Pestos; Root Vegetables; Legumes; Whole Grains; Wild Salmon; Nuts and Seeds; Desserts, Snacks, and Superfoods; and Drinks. You may choose to learn from the book by starting at the beginning and going step by step through the food categories, or you might focus on the foods you're most interested in learning how to cook.

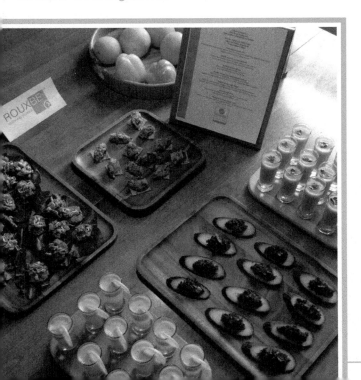

It has been such a joy to create for you this intuitive cooking book with real whole foods. I now invite you to head to a farmers' market, step into your kitchen, and have fun learning simple culinary techniques, intuitively creating meals with whole foods that are available in your market with the season.

Enjoy food & life!

Melanie A. Albert
Phoenix

Philosophies: A New View of Healthy Eating

A new view of healthy eating begins with the food we choose to eat and extends to our shopping, cooking, and eating experiences.

The key philosophies are:

- Eat real whole foods.
- Shop local and in season.
- Enjoy intuitive shopping.
- Cook with intuition.
- Eat mindfully.
- Enjoy food and life.

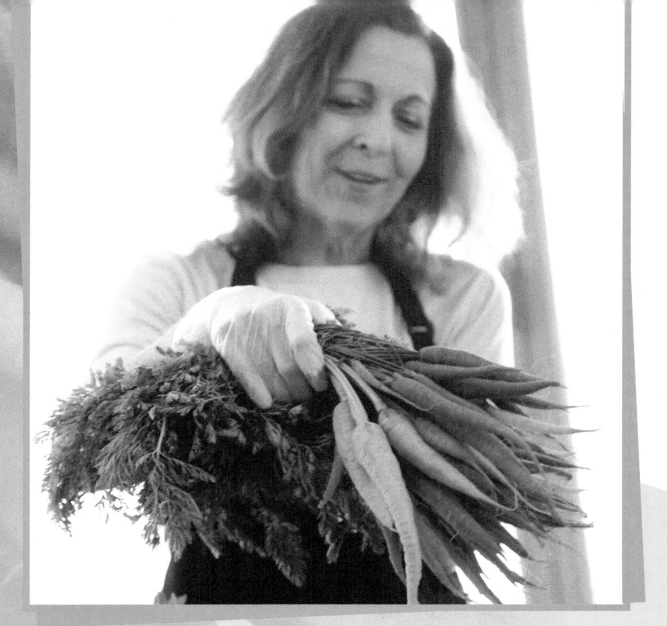

PHILOSOPHIES
A NEW VIEW OF HEALTHY EATING

Eat Real Whole Foods

Eat foods that are in their natural form, as nature created them. Focus on plants and local, in-season foods. Focus on organic. When we eat real whole foods, we get more nutrition and fiber from the foods and receive the energy from the Earth. When we focus on eating organic, we eat food that is "clean," without pesticides or herbicides, and not genetically modified (i.e., not GMO).

Real whole foods include vegetables, fruit, whole grains, legumes, nuts and seeds, and wild salmon. It's quite simple. The recommended foods in "A New View of Healthy Eating" are primarily in alignment with an anti-inflammatory way of eating as advocated by Andrew Weil, M.D., the Mediterranean way of eating, and the Blue Zones as researched by National Geographic, Dan Buettner, and his team. The foods and recipes are all gluten-free and dairy-free.

❝ Real whole foods are real. Think actual vegetables, fruit, grains in their whole form, like brown rice, legumes such as garbanzo beans or lentils, nuts and seeds, and wild cold-water fish like wild salmon. ❞

Shop Local and in Season

When we eat food grown by local farmers, community gardens, or our home gardens, our food is fresher and more nutritious because it has been recently harvested and has not traveled thousands of miles and many days to arrive at a grocery store and our tables. When we eat with the seasons, we eat food that our bodies naturally need at that particular time of the year or location around the world. We also support our local farmers and local economy and have the opportunity to experiment with new, interesting foods.

❝ I love the opportunity to try unique, new-to-me foods, especially when I shop at farmers' markets or receive unfamiliar foods in my CSA (Community Supported Agriculture). I don't always recognize a plant food, but I buy it and experiment in my kitchen or cooking classes. ❞

Enjoy Intuitive Shopping

When we shop for our food, it's important first to pause and listen to our bodies. What are we craving right now? When shopping, mindfully pay attention to the foods, colors, textures, and even aromas you are intuitively attracted to. Sometimes you might be drawn to lots of greens, while other times it may be citrus or tomatoes. It's especially fun to shop at different farmers' markets and notice our choices in food during various seasons of the year.

❝ Intuitive shopping is fun. Listen to your cravings and shop with all your senses. ❞

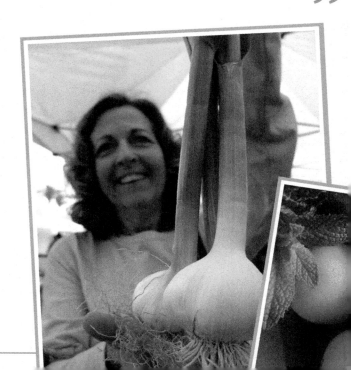

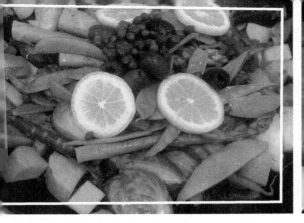
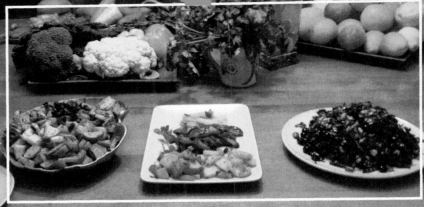

Cook with Intuition

With intuitive cooking, we use recipes as guides. We first learn simple, basic culinary methods and techniques (such as raw, steaming, or roasting) to prepare real whole foods with recipes as our guide. Naturally, over time, we learn to trust our own intuition to cook foods we desire using cooking techniques we've learned. Over time, you will not need to rely on recipes; you'll trust yourself and your culinary skills to create your own healthy dishes with local, seasonal food.

For instance, we learn the culinary technique to steam carrots in a bamboo steamer and use our recipe to finish the carrots with walnut oil, toasted cumin seeds, fresh lemon juice, parsley, and a pinch of sea salt. After learning the bamboo steamer technique to quickly steam veggies, we cook other steamed vegetables (such as asparagus, broccoli, cauliflower, and peapods) and finish them with different oils, spices, and fresh herbs.

> *With intuitive cooking we also naturally cook more mindfully, meditatively enjoying the hythm of chopping veggies or the mindfulness of massaging kale or grating fresh spices.*

Eat Mindfully

When we eat, this is the time to mindfully enjoy our food and its beauty, and to enjoy our family and friends in a beautiful environment. Enjoy the social time to connect with your family or friends. Or, if eating alone, take the time to pause and enjoy the quiet, meditative time for yourself. Set your table with a pleasing environment, using real plates and silverware and perhaps flowers and music. When you eat, pause and enjoy the beauty and aroma of the food grown and lovingly prepared for you. Mindfully eat. Pause, chew, set down your fork, and pause again. Enjoy your meal with all your senses.

> *The key to mindful eating is to pause and enjoy your food and the connections with yourself, your family, and friends.*

Enjoy Food and Life

Food affects life and life affects food. We all make many decisions every day, week, month, year, decade, and life around the foods we eat. Naturally, food affects our bodies and our lives. Food affects our emotions, how our bodies feel, our energy levels, and our self-esteem. And, when we think about it, what's going on in our lives – work, relationships, physical activity, and self-care – all affect our food choices. When we're happier with what's going on in our lives, we naturally make "better" food choices. Of course, the opposite also holds true.

> *The ultimate goal is to embrace and enjoy food and live the life of our dreams.*

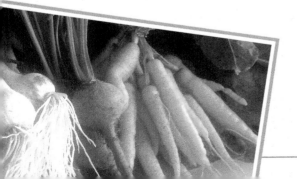

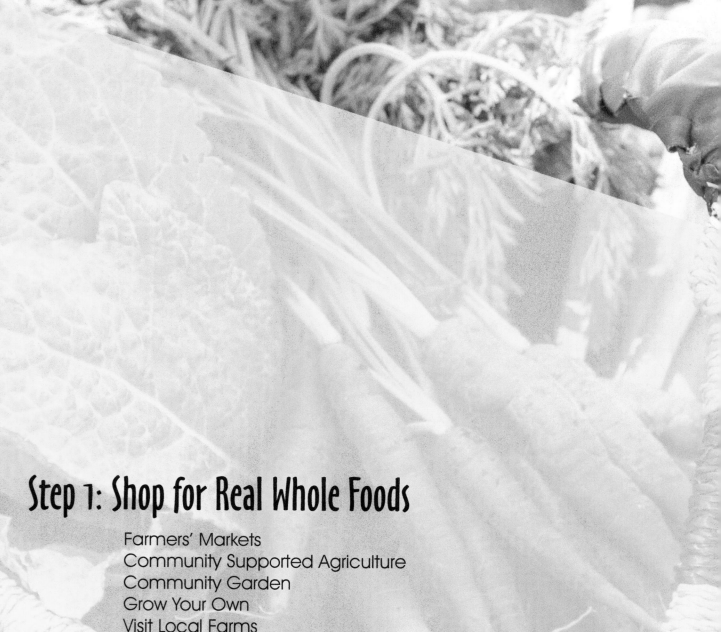

Step 1: Shop for Real Whole Foods

Farmers' Markets
Community Supported Agriculture
Community Garden
Grow Your Own
Visit Local Farms
Eat Organic, Say No to GMO

Step 2: Get your Kitchen Ready for Success

Kitchen Tools
Refrigerator Ready
Pantry
Mise en Place
Recipes

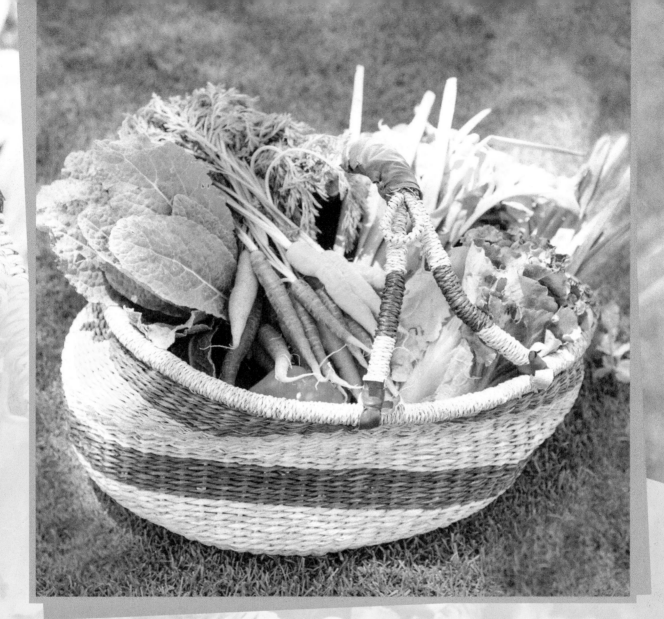

GET SET FOR
HEALTHY EATING SUCCESS

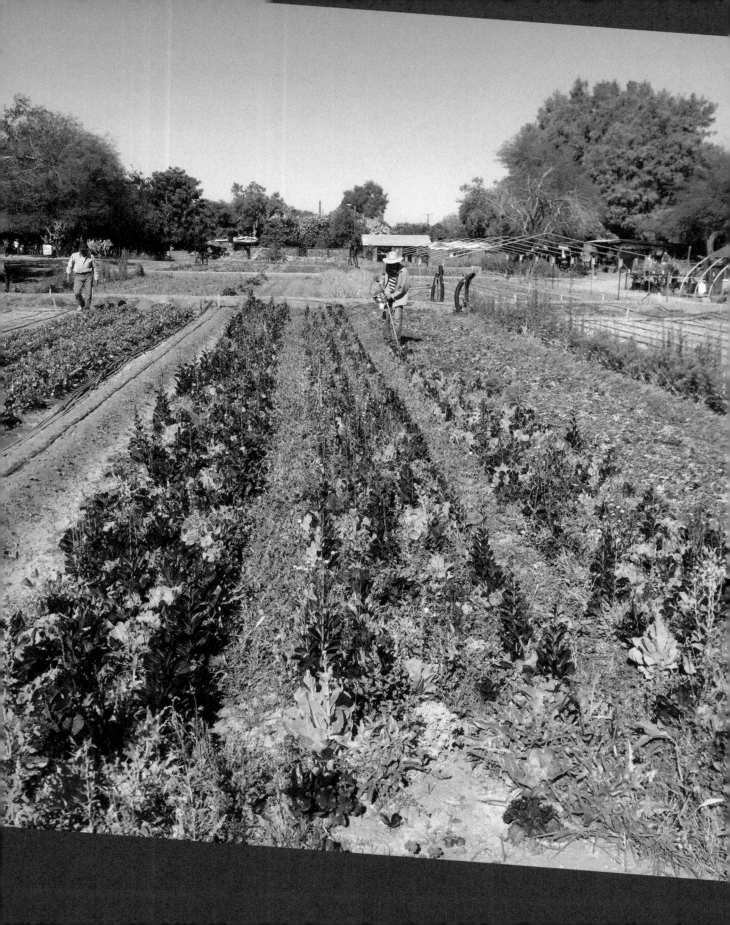

GET SET FOR HEALTHY EATING SUCCESS

Step 1: Shop for Real Whole Foods

Getting set for healthy eating success starts with the food we have available in our homes. We have wonderful options for purchasing fresh, seasonal food so that our kitchens are always ready—stocked with real whole foods to create simple, delicious, healthy meals for ourselves, our families, and our friends. It all starts with the food.

Best Ways to Shop for Real Whole Foods

1. Shop at farmers' markets
2. Commit to a CSA (Community Supported Agriculture) share
3. Join a community garden
4. Grow your own
5. Visit local farms

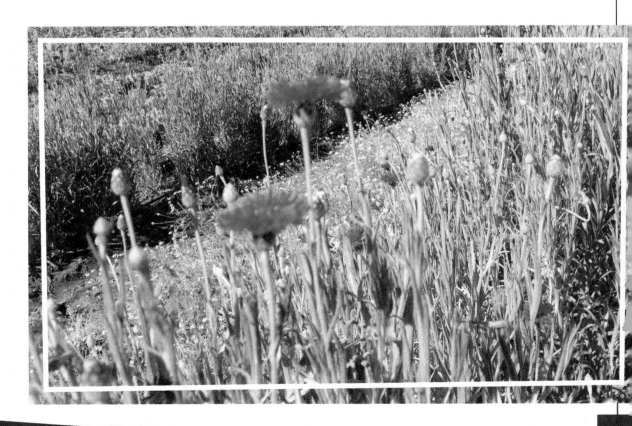

5 BEST WAYS TO SHOP FOR REAL WHOLE FOODS

1. Shop at Farmers' Markets in Your Area

As demand for locally grown fruit and vegetables has increased, farmers' markets have steadily grown in number throughout the last few decades. According to the USDA Farmers Market Directory, in June 2015 there were 8,260 registered farmers' markets as compared to 1,744 in 1994—an increase of more than 6,000 in 21 years. In addition to the USDA Farmers Market Database, another source to find farmers' markets in your area is www.localharvest.org.

2. Commit to a CSA (Community Supported Agriculture) Share

Developed in the 1960's in Japan, CSA programs are designed to build a relationship between the farmer and the community. At the beginning of each season, farmers sell CSA memberships to consumers. Each week, customers receive a sampling of produce that is available from one farmer or a group of local farmers. CSAs cost $25 to $35 per week for six to eight weeks and are perfect for those of us who wish to experiment with unique, interesting, locally grown food. Farmers distribute CSA's at farms, farmers' markets, and convenient pick-up locations, such as yoga studios. Some farms even deliver CSA's right to your home.

For the winter 2016 season in Arizona, I committed to a 12-week CSA share from Maya's Farm, just a mile from my home in Phoenix. I love knowing that the produce is fresh since it is harvested the day before I pick it up at The Farm at South Mountain. Each week the interesting variety of goodies in my CSA encourages me to create new, intuitive dishes with different combinations of food.

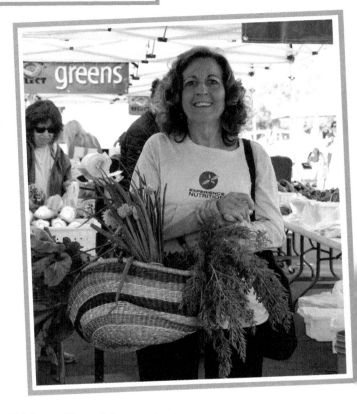

While writing this week, I'm creating a stir-fry with cauliflower, fresh peas, white icicle radish, green garlic, onions, and dill. Fresh flowers are a nice bonus I receive in my CSA. I'm enjoying the incredible natural aromatherapy of chamomile in my home. I'm steeping sun-dried tea, and I will dehydrate some of the chamomile flowers for tea.

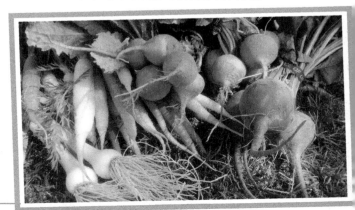

3. Join a Community Garden

The National Garden Association estimates that there are three million community gardens in the United States. Community gardens are fun, as you can learn from other do-it-yourself gardeners, enjoy friendships, and experience the mindful meditation of gardening in a beautiful, close-to-the-earth setting.

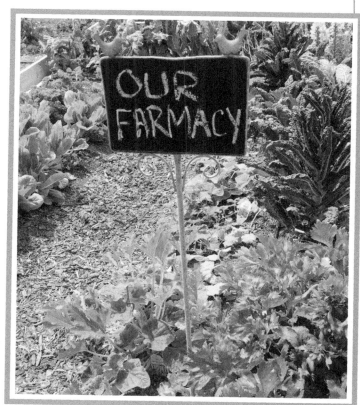

4. Grow Your Own

Gardening is a big trend. As more and more people eat real whole foods, they are taking their food literally into their hands. The National Garden Association estimates that 42 million households in the United States garden, an increase of 17 percent over 2008 numbers, and 37 million households are home gardening. Gardening takes us back to the basics of eating fresh whole foods.

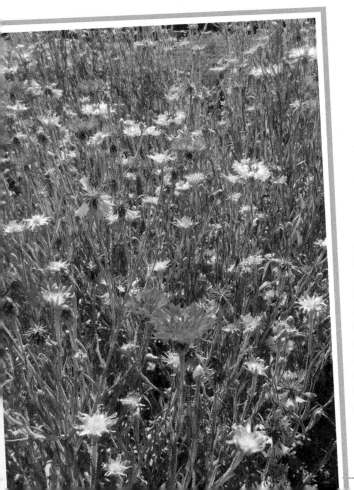

5. Visit Local Farms

It's a lot of fun to visit farms in your area to get to know the farmers and to see where your local produce grows. I am so fortunate that there are many outstanding farms in the Phoenix area, where I live. Farms today are reaching consumers in exciting ways: stores at farms, farmers' markets at farms, pick-your-own produce, and even "honor system" farm stands.

Stores at Farms

In the summer of 2015, I had the honor of presenting a hands-on cooking workshop at a retreat in Scottsdale, Arizona for the Parkinson's Wellness Recovery non-profit organization based in Tucson. Part of the interactive, hands-on workshop included guiding groups of 88 and 80 retreat participants in preparing a raw kale salad. For groups of this size, I needed a case (24 bunches) of kale each week. Because I love the organic dinosaur kale from Blue Sky Farms in Litchfield Park, Arizona, I called to see if I could purchase directly from them. As it turned out, in addition to the farm's business with grocery stores and restaurants, Blue Sky Farms sells to the public in a store right at the farm. It was exciting for my clients and for me that the farmers at Blue Sky Farms went to the field and harvested the kale an hour before I arrived to pick it up, which was 24 hours before my clients created their raw kale salads. Creating salads with just-harvested, fresh, organic kale was a very memorable eat-local-and-with-the-season experience.

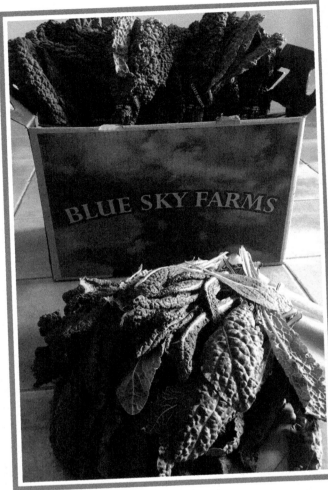

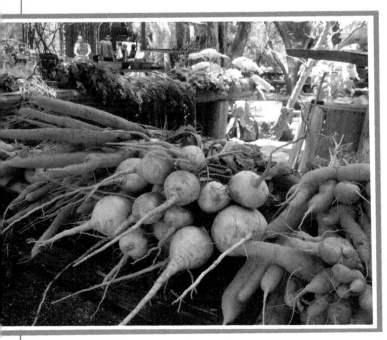

Farmers' Markets at Farms

Another farm, Singh Farms, in Scottsdale, holds a farmers' market on its farm property. This farm is a destination for whole food fun. The farm, a beautiful oasis in the desert, features beautifully displayed, farm-fresh produce under a canopy of trees in the middle of the farm itself. When I visited Singh Farms, they offered other fabulous foods as well, including pizza with corn and basil, wood-cooked corn on the cob, and fresh juice. I enjoyed self-care by being present amid the natural aromatherapy of celery growing right in the middle of the farm in a calm, beautiful environment.

Pick Your Own

Schnepf Farms in Queen Creek, Arizona is a "you-pick-it" farm, with a U-Pick Organic Garden. It's fun to go into the field to harvest veggies right out of the soil and into the orchard to pick peaches. Across the United States, there are many "pick-your-own" farms with seasonal apples, blueberries, and strawberries. Find a "pick-your-own" in your area at www.pickyourown.org.

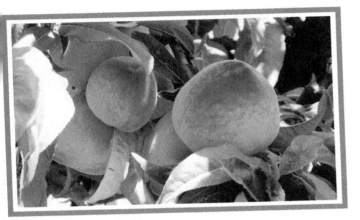

Farm Stands

I grew up shopping at farm stands on the eastern shore of Maryland and I remember eating fresh-picked, juicy tomatoes and sweet corn on the cob. In Arizona, on my drive home from Sedona, I love to shop at a roadside farm stand in Cottonwood because the farmer allows me to get my hands dirty and harvest my produce, including huge onions.

A unique farm stand concept is at The Farm at Agritopia, in Gilbert, Arizona. In addition to selling organic produce at farmers' markets, this small farm has an "honor system" 24-hour self-service farm stand. At this farm stand, you choose your organic produce and purchase it by putting your payment into a little envelope and slot. The honor system concept takes us back to the farm stands of decades past

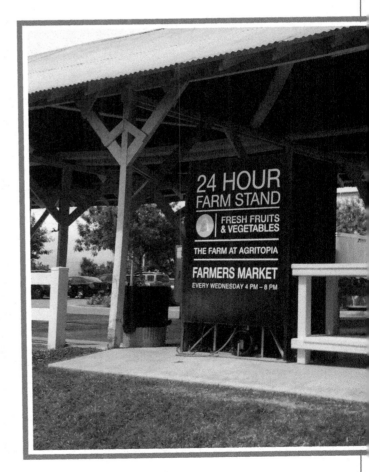

6 Reasons to Eat Local, Seasonal Food

1. **It's more nutritious.** Local produce has a higher nutrition density because we consume it closer to when it was harvested.

2. **You can be in touch with the seasons.** When we eat with the season, foods are at their peak taste and are most abundant. Foods that grow during a particular season and in a particular climate are generally what our bodies need at that time of year. For instance, in hot summers much local produce—such as watermelons, strawberries, and tomatoes—is water-rich and cooling.

3. **The food is farm-fresh.** It tastes better, is fresher, and lasts longer. Produce is just-picked and does not travel 1,500 to 3,000 miles across the United States or from another country.

4. **You can experiment with food.** Have fun cooking different types of food throughout the growing season. Try new veggies, such as striped beets, rainbow carrots, dates, greens, and radishes.

5. **It supports the local economy.** Financially support local farmers in your community by shopping at local farmers' markets or buying a CSA.

6. **It's better for the environment.** There's no need to ship long distances, which lowers the food carbon footprint.

EAT ORGANIC, SAY NO TO GMO

Eating organic is important for our health and our environment. In this section, you will learn how to shop for organic food; you will also learn which foods you must buy organic. In addition, you will get clear on GMOs (genetically modified organisms).

Get Clear on Organic

I've been eating organic food for several decades, way before it became trendy in the news and somewhat mainstream. To me, it made intuitive sense to eliminate pesticides and herbicides from my body and to stay away from genetically modified organisms (GMOs). Years ago it was extremely challenging to shop for organic food. I was able to find organic food, often with limited options, only at small co-ops, such as the Sunseed Natural Foods Co-op, founded in 1974 in Cape Canaveral, Florida. I'm excited that there are so many more shopping options to buy organic across the country and in Phoenix, where I live. I love shopping and supporting local farmers' markets and Arizona farms, many of which grow without pesticides and herbicides. In addition, I love shopping for, cooking with, and eating beautiful, delicious, local, in-season produce.

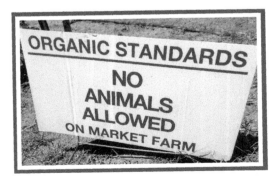

❝ A simple shopping tip: when we eat organic food, by definition we are NOT eating GMOs. So eat organic! **❞**

Get Clear on GMO Produce

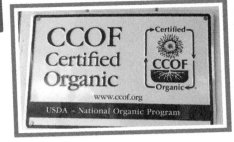

GMOs are rarely in the produce section of grocery stores. Field corn, which is primarily (88 percent of the U.S. crop in 2011) produced with genetically modified seeds, is used to make tortillas, chips, corn syrup, animal feed, and biofuels. Soy, another heavily GMO crop (94 percent of the U.S. crop in 2011), is found in many processed foods.

The genetically modified crops likely to be found in grocery stores in the U.S. are zucchini, yellow squash, Hawaiian papaya, and some varieties of sweet corn.

Since U.S. law does not require the labeling of GMO produce, I recommend purchasing organically grown versions of these foods.

Official USDA Definition of Organic

"Organic food is produced by farmers who emphasize the use of renewable resources and the conservation of soil and water to enhance environmental quality for future generations. Organic meat, poultry, eggs, and dairy products come from animals that are given no antibiotics or growth hormones. Organic food is produced without using most conventional pesticides; fertilizers made with synthetic ingredients or sewage sludge; bioengineering; or ionizing radiation."

Quick Guide: What does organic mean?

The important aspects of organic, as defined by the USDA National Organic Program are:

- No synthetic chemicals or fertilizers
- Not genetically engineered
- Not sterilized by irradiation
- Not fertilized by sewage sludge

Look for the 9!

Stickers or labels attached to fruit and vegetables have a greater function than registering the price at checkout. The PLU (Price Look-Up) code printed on the sticker also tells you how the fruit was grown. By reading the PLU code, you can tell whether the fruit was organically or conventionally grown.

Four numbers in the PLU code: Conventionally or "traditionally" grown with the use of pesticides

PLU code that starts with 9 and has five numbers: Organic and non-GMO

" I'm looking for the 9! Melanie taught me about the importance of eating organic produce, especially those fruits and vegetables which have the most pesticides when conventionally grown. So now when I shop, I'm going to look for 9 as the first number on the small label, as it indicates that the produce is organic. If you see a 4, it's conventionally grown. NFL wife, Ericka Lassiter. "

Dirty Dozen™: Always Buy These Organics

The Dirty Dozen, compiled by the Environmental Working Group, is a list of produce with the highest level of pesticides when conventionally grown. We can lower our pesticide intake substantially by avoiding the 12 most contaminated fruits and vegetables and by eating the least contaminated produce.

Strawberries	Spinach
Apples	Tomatoes
Nectarines	Sweet bell peppers
Peaches	Cherry tomatoes
Celery	Cucumbers
Grapes	Plus: Hot Peppers, Kale/
Cherries	Collard Greens

Which produce has the most pesticides?

Shopper's Guide to Pesticides in Produce

An excellent resource to help us make choices about organic eating is the Handy Shopper's Guide from the non-profit Environmental Working Group (www.EWG.org). This guide tells us which fruits and vegetables have the most pesticide residues and which are the most important to buy organic. The 2016 guide ranks the pesticide contamination of 48 popular fruits and vegetables based on an analysis of more than 35,200 samples taken by the USDA and FDA. The USDA doesn't test every food every year, so the EWG uses the most recent sampling period for each type of food.

The Shopper's Guide to Pesticides in Produce is aware that some people who wish to reduce their exposure to pesticides cannot always find or afford to eat organic produce. The guide helps them seek out conventionally grown fruits and vegetables that tend to test low for pesticide residue (Clean Fifteen™). When we want to purchase produce whose conventional versions test high for pesticides (Dirty Dozen™), we can make an effort to locate organic versions.

The Clean Fifteen™: Produce with the Lowest Pesticide Residues, OK to Eat Conventionally Grown

EWG's Clean Fifteen™ is a list of produce which are least likely to hold pesticide residues. Relatively few pesticides were detected on these foods, and tests found low total concentrations of pesticides on them. If you are on a budget or cannot find organic versions of these fruits and vegetables, use this guide as a resource to purchase produce with the lowest levels of pesticides.

Avocados	Onions	Honeydew
Sweet corn	Asparagus	Melon
Pineapples	Mangos	Grapefruit
Cabbage	Papayas	Cantaloupe
Sweet peas	Kiwi	Cauliflower
frozen	Eggplant	

 Action

Now that you have learned about shopping options for local, seasonal produce and the meaning of organic and GMO, I invite you to visit a farm or farmers' market in your area and shop for food that looks interesting to you. Have fun!

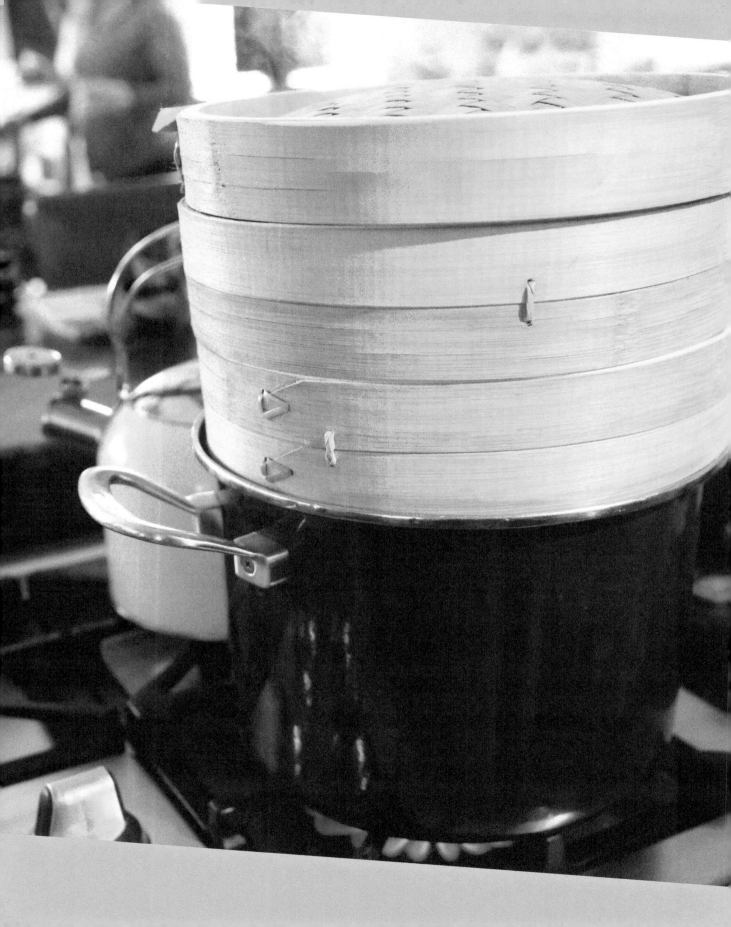

Step 2: Kitchen

To create healthy meals at home, you must stock your kitchen with basic tools and your refrigerator and pantry with healthy staples. Mindful cooking requires organization. You'll develop a new view of healthy eating as you use recipes to discover simple, basic culinary techniques and then intuitively create your own dishes.

5 Vital Steps to Get Your Kitchen Ready for Healthy Eating Success

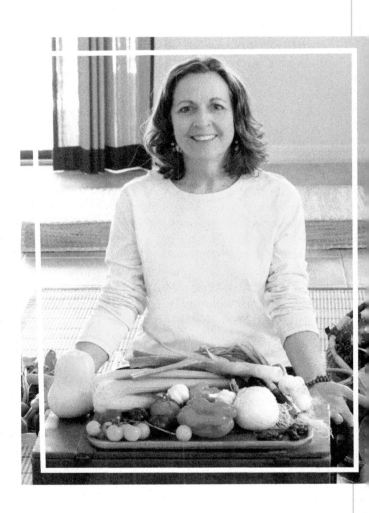

1. **Kitchen Tools.** Basic kitchen tools to cook simple, easy-to-prepare whole food creations.
2. **Refrigerator Ready.** Key staples and foods to always have in your refrigerator, to be ready to cook simple whole food meals.
3. **Pantry.** Be prepared with staples to cook with what's in season and what you bring home from the farmers' market.
4. **Mise en Place.** How to be organized when you cook for efficiency and mindfulness in the kitchen.
5. **Recipes.** Learn basic culinary techniques and use recipes as guides; then intuitively create your own dishes.

5 VITAL STEPS TO GET YOUR KITCHEN READY FOR HEALTHY EATING SUCCESS

Step 1: Kitchen Tools

When we think about kitchen tools, it's important to consider the basic equipment we need in a kitchen to cook simple and healthy meals, desserts, and beverages. With a few essential tools, your cooking experience will be easier and more enjoyable. While discussing the basic tools for our kitchens, it makes sense to consider the different ways we will be preparing and cooking food: raw, steaming, sautéing, roasting, and baking.

In reality, we need only a very few tools for all cooking: a knife, a cutting board, wooden spoons, a sauté pan, a soup pot, a bamboo steamer, a rice cooker, a flat baking sheet, a food processor, and a high-speed blender. We also need a few small items, including glass jars, a spiralizer, and natural parchment paper. Plus, a dehydrator for raw food preparation is a nice addition.

❝ When traveling for a week or more, I take my favorite Chef knife with me, as it is so much nicer to cook with 'my' knife that fits 'just right' in my hand; it cuts food smoothly. **❞**

Knife

A knife that is "right for you" is the number-one most valuable kitchen tool. The key aspects of a knife are: fits comfortably in your hand, feels balanced, and is sharp. For me, a basic Chef's knife, 6-inch or 8-inch, can be used for virtually all cutting in the kitchen. Before you purchase a knife, visit a kitchen store and experiment by holding and cutting with different knives to determine which works best for you.

Some people prefer stainless steel, relatively heavy German knives. Others prefer lighter, thin Japanese knives, while still others prefer lightweight, colored ceramic knives. The most important thing is to find a knife that feels comfortable in your hand and to know that the investment is worth it, as each of us tends to use our favorite knife every day, for years and even decades.

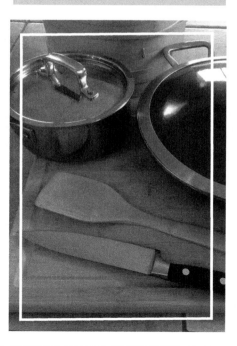

Bamboo Cutting Board

Cutting boards are essential in the kitchen to make cutting easier with a flat surface, protect your kitchen counters, and keep knives sharp. My favorite cutting boards are made of bamboo, as they are clean, sustainable, and naturally anti-bacterial and anti-microbial. Cutting boards last decades, so finding the right cutting board to invest in is important. A key to purchasing a cutting board is to be sure that it is large enough that your entire knife (blade and handle) stays within the board when you chop.

Wooden Spoons

A few wooden spoons are staples in the kitchen and are used to move food around in a sauté pan or to stir food in a pot. Personally, I prefer bamboo with a flat edge. Bamboo, a grass, grows at a fast rate, so it is eco-friendly and biodegradable. It's strong and durable, and will not scratch cookware

Sauté Pan

An 8- to 10-inch sauté pan is essential for stove-top cooking. My favorite sauté pans are enamel and stainless steel, which are both non-stick. I use them a few times a week to sauté veggies and often to make tomato sauce.

Large Soup Pot

For cooking soups, beans, and sauces, a heavy 6- to 8-quart pot is a must. I love my Chantal Copper Fusion 8-Quart pot, which heats and cooks quickly.

Flat Baking Sheet

Most people call these cookie sheets. I use a heavy, flat, stainless steel baking sheet with a high rim for roasting veggies and melting chocolate chips. An 18-inch by 13-inch baking sheet works well for everyday use.

High-Speed Blender

A quality blender is a must for smoothies and having fun with raw cooking, as it provides optimal consistency and smoothness. Use high-speed blenders for nut-based creams, sauces, soups, dressings, soft nut-based cheeses, non-dairy milk, smoothies, and cracking whole grains.

" I love my Chantal Copper Fusion 11½-Inch, 3-Quart Chef Pan that cooks food quickly and evenly. Veggies stay vibrant and bright when cooked in this pan. Fused copper provides excellent, even heat distribution over the entire cooking surface. The enamel surface is naturally stick-resistant. "

Bamboo Steamer

For simple, quick veggie cooking, a bamboo steamer is a low-cost kitchen tool essential. A 10-inch steamer with two levels is perfect. Be sure to have a large pot for the steamer to sit above boiling water.

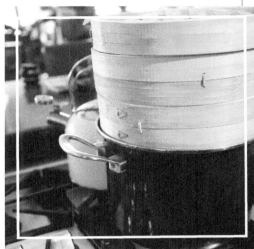

Rice Cooker

For a very easy way to cook brown rice and other whole grains, a simple rice cooker is an excellent addition to the kitchen. If you do not have a rice cooker, a 3-quart pot is perfect for cooking a cup of grains.

Food Processor

A basic food processor is an important kitchen tool to mix and blend ingredients. Food processors blend thick creams and sauces; chop veggies, nuts, and seeds; create nut butter; and are used to make many snacks and desserts.

" Invest in a quality food processor. My food processor is 25 years old and still works just fine. "

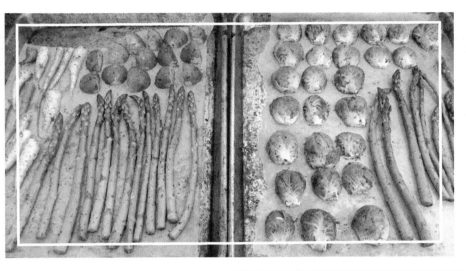

Spiralizer

A spiral veggie slicer is a simple hand-held machine that very easily turns vegetables such as zucchini, sweet potatoes, butternut squash, and beets into noodle-like shapes. Veggie noodles are perfect in raw salads or sautéed side dishes.

Glass Jars

Glass jars are used in several different ways in a whole food kitchen, including for storing nuts, seeds, grains and beans; shaking homemade salad dressing; and sprouting beans and whole grains. In my kitchen, I use quart and pint glass jars.

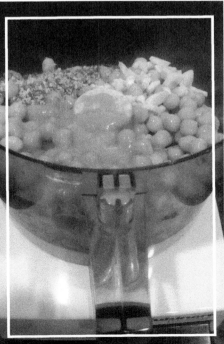

Parchment Paper

Used on the flat baking sheet for crispy roasted veggies and easier clean-up. Unbleached parchment paper is unbleached, chlorine-free, and compostable.

Step 2:
Refrigerator Ready

Get your refrigerator ready for healthy eating success. To be prepared to cook simple meals with real whole foods, it is important to have our refrigerators ready with a few basic real whole foods and staples. That way, whenever we are cooking, we have the staple ingredients to create a meal. Thus, we are more likely to create a quick, simple, healthy meal.

New Way of Shopping

Shop for the basics at your local farmers' market, natural grocery store, or co-op and keep these in your refrigerator and pantry year-round. When you always have the staple foods in your refrigerator, it's fun to shop at farmers' markets to creatively add to the basics. While shopping, pay attention to your desires and cravings, listen to your body and heart, and intuitively choose colorful, texture-rich, or aromatic foods that appeal to you.

" When I shop for my own personal cooking, cooking classes, and events, I start with local Arizona farmers' markets and then fill in the gaps with natural foods stores. **"**

6 Everyday Veggies

Stock your kitchen with a few basic vegetables to use all the time in quick salads, roasted veggies, steamed veggies, or smoothies, or juicing.

1. Avocados
2. Tomatoes
3. Sweet potatoes
4. Carrots or other roots such as beets
5. Kale or other leafy greens such as collard greens
6. Celery

5 Essential Everyday Fruit

Always have several types of fruit in your refrigerator; use citrus in salad dressings, berries in smoothies, and apples as a quick snack.

1. Lemons
2. Limes
3. Oranges
4. Apples
5. Berries (fresh or frozen), such as raspberries or blueberries

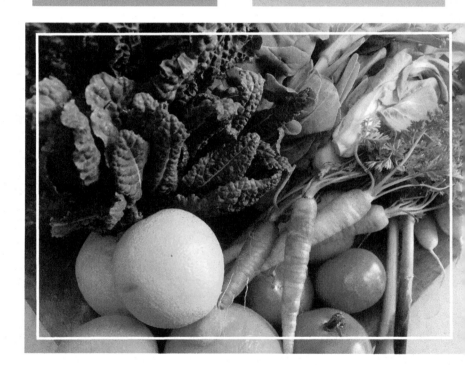

4 Basic Fresh Herbs and Spices

Keep a few fresh herbs (basil, parsley, cilantro) stored in a cup of fresh water in your refrigerator to add flavor to food creations, including avocado salsa, hummus, salads, and nut pâtés. Fresh ginger root, a power anti-inflammatory, is perfect for salad dressings, veggie stir-fries, and smoothies.

2 Favorite Aromatics

Keep at least two aromatics (onions, fresh garlic) in your kitchen to add flavor to cooked and raw food.

Step 3: Pantry: Essentials in the Whole Food Pantry

Stock your pantry with essentials so that you are prepared to cook with seasonal food you bring home from the farmers' market. With these essentials, you can intuitively create your own favorite dishes for breakfast, lunch, dinner, or snacks.

Whole grains

Use versatile whole grains such as brown rice, quinoa, and steel-cut oats to quickly and simply cook breakfast with berries, nuts, and seeds, or a dinner side dish with raw, steamed, or roasted vegetables.

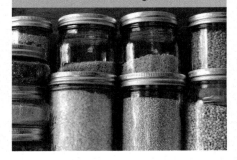

Beans and legumes

Cook garbanzo beans for a quick hummus, lentils in a simple soup, adzuki beans for a simple rice and beans meal, and kidney beans in a veggie chili.

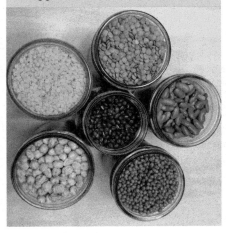

Nuts and seeds

Enjoy a variety of nuts and seeds such as almonds, cashews, walnuts, hemp seeds, and sunflower seeds. Blend nut milk, add to smoothies, cook in a stir-fry, or make a raw pâté.

Extra virgin olive oil

Buy organic, first press, cold press, estate grown, and with <.8 acidity for a high-quality olive oil. Olive oil is perfect for salad dressings, roasting veggies, finishing steamed vegetables, and dipping flatbread.

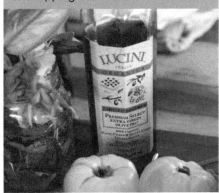

Dried herbs and spices

Stock a few dried herbs (basil, oregano, marjoram, bay leaves) and spices (cumin seeds, coriander, cinnamon) in your pantry. Use a few different spices and herbs every week to intuitively add flavor and dimension to roasted roots, baked spaghetti squash, and hummus.

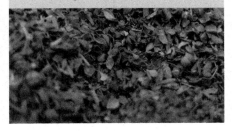

Vinegar and mustard

Keep a few acids, such as balsamic, red wine, or rice vinegar, and stone-ground mustard in your pantry for salad and vegetable dressings and marinades. There's always an 18-year aged balsamic vinegar in my pantry that I love to drizzle on roasted veggies and that I use as a dipping sauce for my organic sprouted flatbread.

Sweeteners

Use natural sweeteners such as fresh Medjool dates and local raw honey in your breakfast whole grains, salad dressings, smoothies, and desserts.

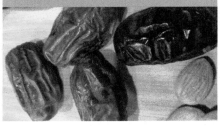

Sea salt

Try a few types of unrefined sea salts such as Celtic or Himalayan salts and cook with those you like best. Sea salt brings out the natural flavor in food. For cooking at home and in my classes and workshops, I love whole crystal (coarse) unrefined salt that sometimes needs a little grinding.

Green tea and coconut water

Use electrolyte-rich coconut water as a base for smoothies, and drink loose green tea and matcha tea as everyday beverages.

A few extras for extra flavor

We all have a few special foods that we love to add to our meals. I often add olives and capers to veggie stir-fries and simple avocado salads.

Superfoods

Stock a few nutrient-dense superfoods, such as goji berries, raw cacao nibs, and hemp seeds for quick snacks or smoothies.

Step 4: Mise en Place: Be Organized When You Cook

Mise en Place (French pronunciation: [mi zã plas] is a French phrase that means "putting in place," as in "setting up."

Mise en Place is used in the kitchen to "set up" all the ingredients needed to prepare a dish before we start cooking. The purpose is to be organized when we cook, with everything ready so that it's easier to cook. Mise en Place is a useful cooking technique to incorporate when you are cooking in your kitchen for both complex and simple recipes.

With the Mise en Place concept, before we start cooking we get all the ingredients ready, sliced, diced, measured, and organized. To be super organized, we can even set up our ingredients in order of use in the cooking process, which is especially beneficial when cooking a fast-paced meal like a stir-fry or a recipe with a lot of ingredients.

4 Reasons to Love Mise en Place

1. **Be prepared and calm.** You will not be scrambling around your kitchen during the middle of the cooking process, looking for that one ingredient you really need. Also, you will be so organized that you won't need to rush out to purchase a missing ingredient.
2. **Cook when cooking.** You will not need to quickly chop food you might have forgotten about right in the middle of the cooking process. You will mindfully enjoy cooking your meal.
3. **Save time.** As an example, if you are mincing onions or garlic for several dishes, you can mince them at the same time while setting up your Mise en Place.
4. **Cook mindfully and clutter-free**. Cooking is much more enjoyable in a neat, clutter-free environment. Your cooking process will be mindful and beautiful when you cook in an organized fashion.

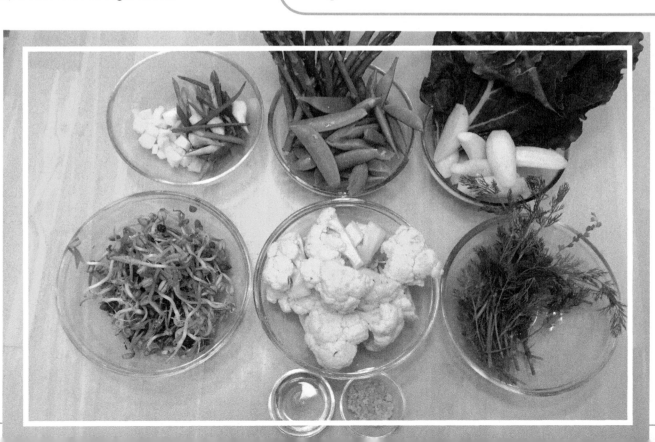

Step 5: Recipes: Learn Basic Culinary Techniques using Recipes as Guides, then Cook Intuitively

With a new way of cooking intuitively for healthy eating, you will learn basic culinary skills and practice simple cooking techniques with simple recipes. With these culinary skills and practice, ultimately you will intuitively cook simple-to-prepare, delicious, beautiful meals with what's seasonally available at the farmers' market and in your refrigerator.

Basic Whole Food Cooking Culinary Skills

You will learn basic culinary techniques such as raw, steaming, sautéing, roasting, broiling, baking, marinating, and finishing. Once learned, you can use these cooking techniques or culinary skills to prepare a variety of dishes and meals.

Learn with Recipes. Then Cook Intuitively

The recipes in this book are designed to teach you how to cook different foods with different cooking techniques and different combinations of food. Once you master the recipes, use your new skills to create your own individualized, creative meals with foods available at your farmers' markets and taking into account your personal food likes, desires, and cravings. With this way of simple, intuitive cooking, recipes become guides; you can substitute ingredients to confidently create your favorite dishes.

Roast Roots

After you learn how to simply roast a root vegetable, such as sweet potatoes with organic extra virgin olive oil, sea salt, and a few dried herbs, transfer your cooking skills to roast other in-season roots, such as golden beets, onions, and colorful radishes.

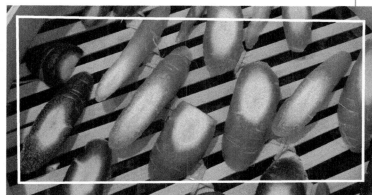

Steam Veggies

Another example is steaming carrots in a bamboo steamer and finishing them with walnut oil, fresh lemon juice, toasted cumin seeds, and sea salt. Once you know how to very quickly steam vegetables in a steamer basket, you can use this culinary skill to steam other vegetables. And once you've learned to finish carrots, use the same method to finish veggies with different oils, herbs, spices, nuts, and seeds.

> **"** Once you learn a few basic cooking techniques and basic recipes, you will have the skills to intuitively cook your favorite foods very easily and with confidence. **"**

 ## Action

In our live cooking classes, participants learn basic culinary skills with specific recipes. Each week they practice their prior learning. In the last class, "no recipe night," participants, in friendly competition, create dishes using the skills they've learned. I invite you to incorporate this way of cooking into your life. Use your new culinary skills and recipes as guides to create your own unique dishes based on your cravings and what's in your refrigerator. Have fun and share your creations with us on Facebook: www.facebook.com/NewViewHealthyEating

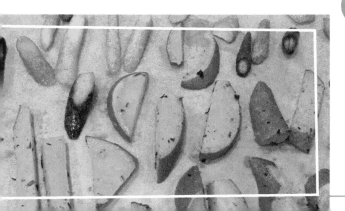

Make Raw Veggies Interesting

Culinary

- Massage raw kale
- Basic salad dressing, with 3 ingredients
- 6 ways to create your own salad dressing
- How to shop for high quality olive oil
- 4 Ways to create your own kale salad
- How to dry toast nuts
- How to spiralize veggies
- Create your own cashew pesto dressing
- Create your own avocado salsa
- Simple steps to grow an avocado tree
- 7 simple ways to enjoy avocados
- How to select the best avocado
- What is dehydrating?
- How to shop for a high quality dehydrator

Recipes

- EXPERIENCE NUTRITION™ Signature Raw Massaged Kale Salad
- Asian Salad with Vibrant Purple Cabbage and Tangy Citrus Ginger Root Dressing
- Raw Cashews & Basil Pesto
- EXPERIENCE NUTRITION™ Signature Avocado Salsa
- Summer Time Tomato Gazpacho Cold Soup
- Kale Chips: Dehydrate or Bake

Nutrition

- Olive oil as an anti-inflammatory
- The power of ginger
- Avocados are a good monounsaturated fat

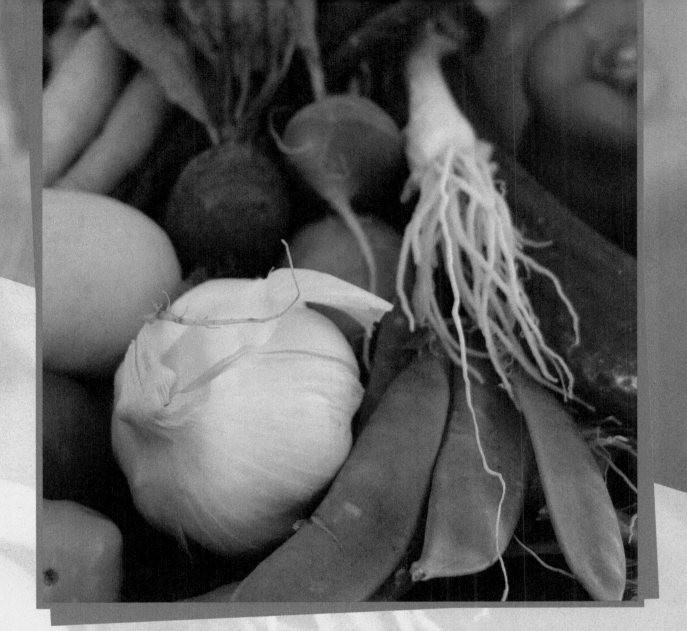

MAKE RAW
VEGGIES INTERESTING

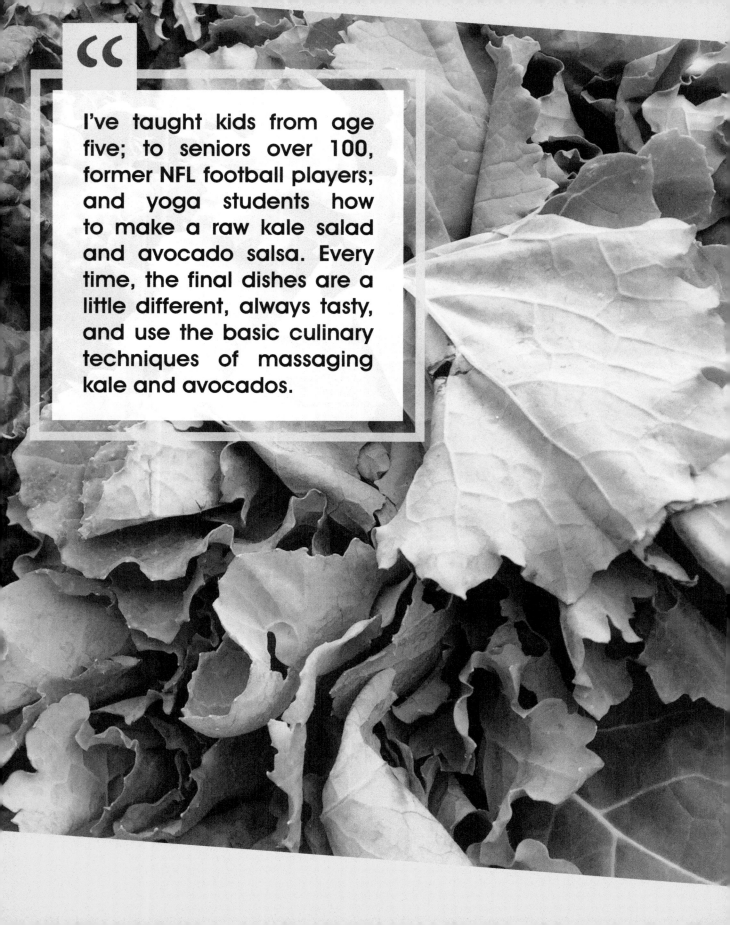

> I've taught kids from age five; to seniors over 100, former NFL football players; and yoga students how to make a raw kale salad and avocado salsa. Every time, the final dishes are a little different, always tasty, and use the basic culinary techniques of massaging kale and avocados.

MAKE RAW VEGGIES INTERESTING

Eating veggies does not need to be boring

Many people think that eating veggies is nothing more than consuming chopped raw carrots and a stalk of celery with a glass of water. Eating raw veggies is so much more than that. While I am not a raw foodist, I do enjoy some veggies raw, especially when the weather is warm and when fresh, water-rich fruit and vegetables are in season. Think watermelon, cucumbers, and tomatoes.

In this section, you'll learn several very simple ways to prepare raw foods and to use them to make healthy, delish, tasty dishes, including the 4 "S's": salads, salsas, soup, and snacks. You'll learn how to:

- Massage kale to break down the fiber and create a tender raw kale salad.
- Intuitively create Asian salad with vibrant purple cabbage and tangy ginger root dressing.
- Create a perfect salad dressing every time with three basic ingredients.
- Spiralize veggies and make a creamy vegan nut-based dressing.
- Create avocado salsa with what's available in the refrigerator.
- Make refreshing cold soup with in-season heirloom tomatoes.
- Dehydrate kale for a crunchy super-food snack.

You'll also learn tips to shop for:

- High-quality olive oil
- The best avocado
- A dehydrator

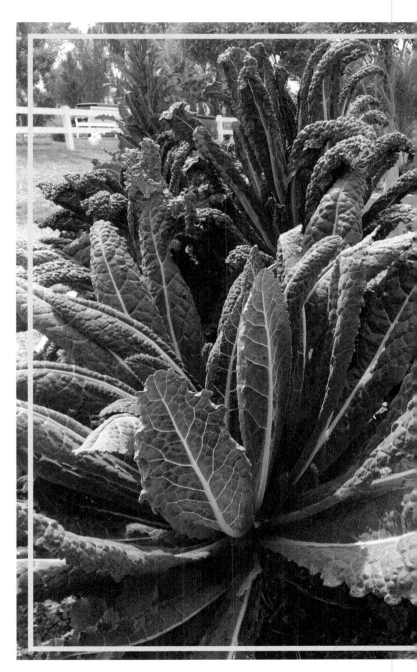

EXPERIENCE NUTRITION™ SIGNATURE RAW MASSAGED KALE SALAD

Make your own gourmet raw kale salad with your favorite fruit, berries, nuts, and seeds. Learn how to make a simple salad dressing, massage your kale, and add your favorite seasonal fruit, berries, nuts, and seeds.

Basic Salad Dressing: 3 Ingredients. That's It

Three base ingredients for a salad dressing include a fat, an acid, and salt. Optional add-ins are aromatics (such as garlic and onions), fresh herbs (like basil and oregano), and sweeteners like local raw honey and fresh dates. To make your first dressing for a kale salad, start with fresh lemon, organic extra virgin olive oil, sea salt, and garlic. Once you've learned how to prepare a dressing with this technique, you can use this method to create your own unique salad dressings for a raw kale salad or other fresh salads.

SIMPLE INGREDIENTS

- 1 fresh lemon, squeezed, approximately ¼ cup juice, approximately ½ cup
- Organic extra virgin olive oil, twice as much as the lemon
- ¼ tsp sea salt
- 2-3 garlic cloves, minced

SIMPLE STEPS

1. Squeeze a fresh organic lemon into a pint-size Mason jar.
2. Pour in twice as much olive oil as the lemon.
3. Sprinkle in sea salt and minced garlic.
4. Shake the jar.
5. Taste and notice if your dressing seems too oily or acid-tasting, or if it uses too little or too much salt. Taste testing salad dressing is a great way to mindfully use your cooking intuition. Add ingredients until the dressing tastes great.

 Ways to Create Your Own Salad Dressing

Learn the simple salad dressing technique and then create your own with different fats, different acids, and various add-ins, such as freshly minced herbs or sweeteners. Use sweeteners to balance a dressing that seems too acid-tasting.

1. **Fats**: Olive oil, grapeseed oil, nut oils such as walnut oil
2. **Acid**: Citrus (lemons, limes, oranges); vinegar (balsamic, rice, red or white wine), or stone-ground mustard
3. **Salt**: Your choice of sea salt or Himalayan salt
4. **Optional Sweeteners**: Raw honey or dates
5. **Optional Aromatics**: Garlic, green onions, shallots, red onions
6. **Optional Freshly Minced Herbs**: Basil, cilantro, oregano, parsley

" The key to a tender kale salad is a simple dressing and massaging the kale. It's fun to create a beautiful, tasty kale salad with seasonal fruit and berries. One of my very favorite add-ins in a kale salad is local Arizona organic pomegranate seeds, which add a sweet, sharp taste and nice crunchiness to the salad. "

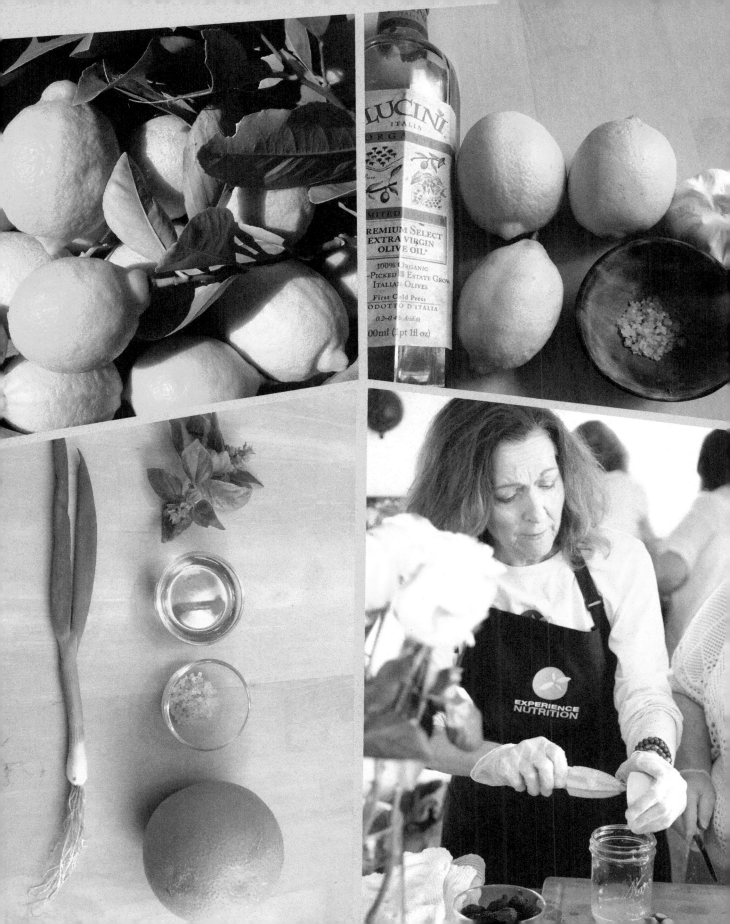

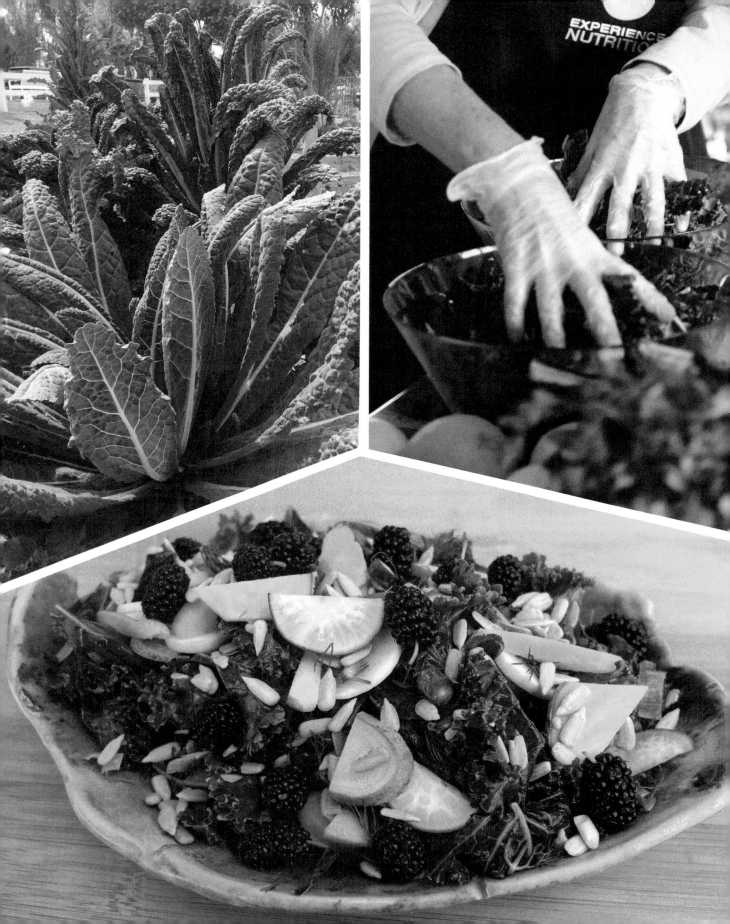

THE RAW KALE SALAD

In addition to fresh homemade dressing, the key to creating an outstanding raw kale salad is massaging the kale. Yes, massaging the kale! When we massage kale, we marinate the leaves and break down the fiber; the kale leaves become tender, soft, and flavorful.

SIMPLE INGREDIENTS

- Bunch of kale: Dinosaur (Lacinato or Tuscan), green curly leafy, dark red (redbor)
- 1 cup strawberries, sliced
- 1 cup blueberries or blackberries
- ¼ cup Mission figs, chopped
- 1 cup seeds, sunflower or pumpkin; raw or dry toasted

SIMPLE STEPS

1. Tear or cut out the fibrous center of kale leaves.
2. Chop or tear kale into bite-size pieces or ribbons.
3. Pour dressing over kale.
4. Massage kale for about 5-7 minutes. Massaging the kale is key. Massage the kale with your hands to marinate it. Do not toss.
5. Add three-quarters of the strawberries, blueberries, Mission figs, and seeds to the kale and gently toss.
6. Sprinkle the remaining berries, figs, and seeds on top of the salad when plating.
7. Enjoy!

5 Ways to Mindfully Create Your Own Kale Salad

Once you have learned how to massage kale, mindfully and intuitively create your own version of a kale salad with different types of kale, in-season fruit and veggies, and raw or toasted nuts and seeds.

1. **Kale:** Dinosaur (Lacinato or Tuscan), green curly leafy, dark red (redbor)
2. **Fruit:** Apples, pears, grapes, pomegranate
3. **Berries:** Blueberries, blackberries, raspberries, strawberries
4. **Roots:** Beets, radishes
5. **Nuts and Seeds:** Almonds, cashews, pumpkin seeds, sunflower seeds, walnuts

" Many of my cooking clients and I love to mindfully massage the kale. It's part of the enjoyable experience in the kitchen. "

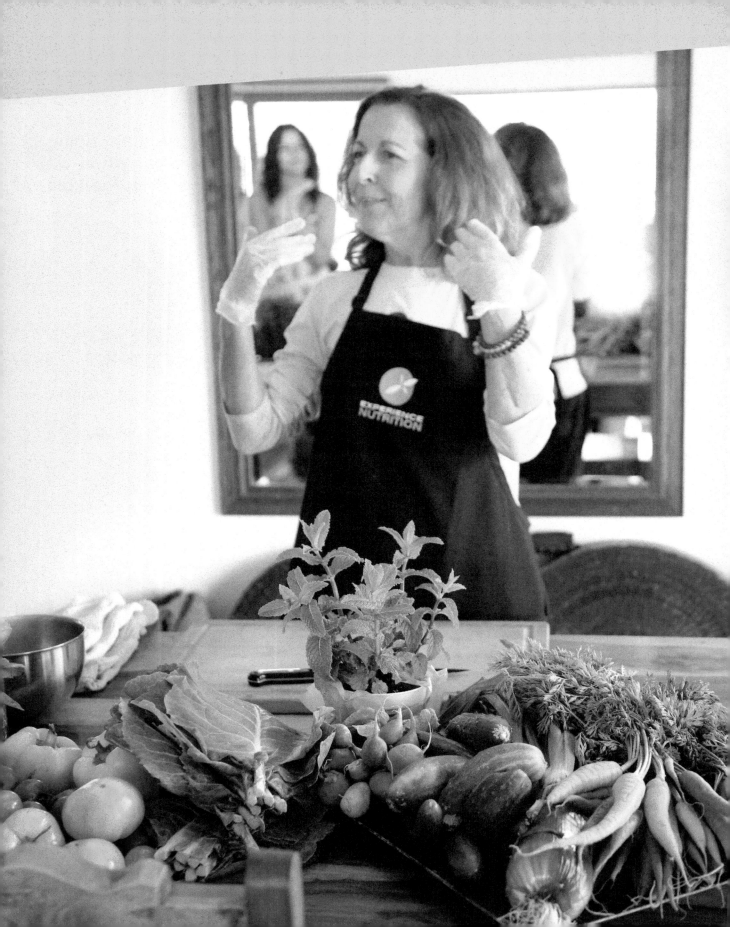

How to Shop for a High-Quality Organic Olive Oil

The International Olive Council (IOC) promotes olive oil around the world by tracking production, defining quality standards, and monitoring authenticity. More than 98 percent of the world's olives grow in IOC member nations. (www.InternationalOliveOil.org)

Olive Oil Terminology

- **Extra virgin olive oil (EVOO)**. The highest quality olive oil, produced by a simple pressing of the olives. It contains no more than 0.8 percent acidity, and is judged to have a superior taste. EVOO accounts for less than 10 percent of oil in many producing countries.

- **Cold Pressed EVOO**. Is not heated above a certain temperature (usually 80 degrees Fahrenheit) during processing; thus, it retains more nutrients and experiences less degradation.

- **First Cold Pressed EVOO**. Comes from olives that have been crushed exactly one time, i.e., the first press. The "cold" refers to the temperature range of the fruit at the time it is crushed.

- **From Hand-Picked Olives**. Implies that the oil is of better quality because producers harvesting olives by mechanical methods are inclined to let olives over-ripen as a means of increasing yield.

Enjoy Olive Oil as an Anti-Inflammatory

Recent research suggests that some premium olive oils that contain a compound called oleocanthal offer anti-inflammatory properties similar to non-steroidal anti-inflammatory drugs like ibuprofen. If you experience a little peppery taste, a sting in your throat, or a cough when you swallow, the olive oil has this healthy compound. This does not mean that a little olive oil once in a while will relieve your pain, but olive oil may provide long-term benefits.

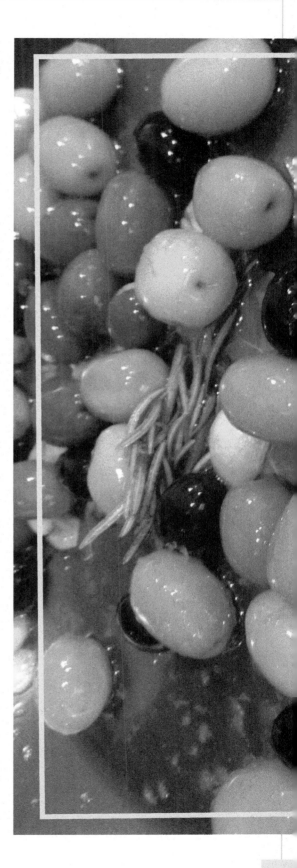

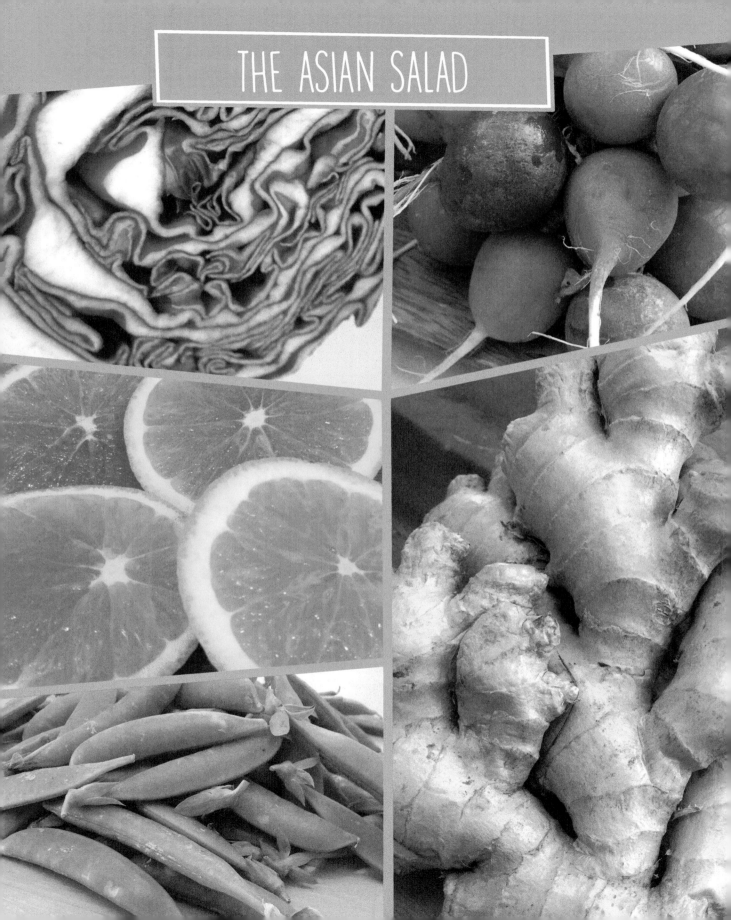

THE ASIAN SALAD

Asian Salad with Vibrant Purple Cabbage and Tangy Citrus Ginger Root Dressing

Make your own gourmet Asian salad with a rainbow of raw organic veggies, your favorite toasted nuts, and intuitively created ginger root dressing.

Asian Salad: Ginger Salad Dressing: 3 Key Ingredients

The essential ingredients for a perfect Asian dressing every time are ginger root, a soy flavoring (wheat-free tamari soy sauce or Bragg's amino acids), and fresh citrus.

SIMPLE INGREDIENTS

- 1" fresh ginger root
- 1 garlic clove, minced
- ½ cup soy tamari or Bragg's amino acids
- ½ orange, juiced
- ½ fresh-squeezed lemon or lime juice
- 1 tbsp rice wine vinegar
- 1 tsp local honey
- ½ cup organic extra virgin olive oil

SIMPLE STEPS

1. Finely mince ginger root and garlic.
2. Place in pint-size Mason jar.
3. Add all other ingredients (except olive oil) to jar and shake.
4. Taste and intuitively add ingredients to create your desired flavor.
   - Too much acid: add olive oil
   - Not sweet enough: add honey
   - Too oily: add lemon or lime juice

The Power of Ginger

Ginger is a tropical plant whose roots have been used medicinally in Asia for centuries. Ginger root is a natural anti-inflammatory; it reduces nausea, helps digestion, and is good for colds and flu. A simple way to add fresh ginger to your food is to use it in a salad dressing.

❝ The key to a delicious ginger root salad dressing is tasting the dressing while you are making it for just the right balance of ginger, citrus, and soy flavor. **❞**

Asian Rainbow Salad

Along with a tangy ginger root dressing, a colorful rainbow of raw organic veggies creates a beautiful Asian salad.

SIMPLE INGREDIENTS

- 1 purple cabbage, shredded
- 2 cups Napa cabbage, shredded
- 1 cup carrots, shredded
- 1 cucumber, julienned (long, thin slices)
- 1 cup snap peas or snow peas, cut on bias
- 6 green onions, cut on bias
- 1 cup red or purple radishes, shredded
- 1 cup almonds, sliced and dry toasted

SIMPLE STEPS

1. Dry toast (no oil) sliced almonds in small sauté pan on low heat for 5 minutes.
2. Toss all vegetables in a large bowl and mix thoroughly.
3. Drizzle the Asian salad dressing on the vegetables and gently toss.
4. Top with dry toasted almonds.
5. Enjoy!

How to Quickly Dry Toast Nuts to Bring out their Nutty Flavor

Heat a small stainless steel sauté pan on low. Add sliced almonds and stir them in the pan for about 5 minutes. Nuts cook very quickly, so be sure to occasionally stir the nuts to prevent them from burning.

❝ We eat with our eyes first. Cut your veggies in different shapes and sizes for visual texture in your salad. **❞**

SPIRAL VEGGIES WITH NUT-BASED CREAMY DRESSING

Learn how to spiral colorful veggies and create a simple dressing with raw cashews and basil.

Basic Salad Dressing: Raw Cashews & Basil Pesto

A vegan, dairy-free, creamy dressing is the base for this colorful raw spiral veggie salad. With fresh basil and lots of garlic, this refreshing dressing is a perfect alternative to a cheese-based pesto.

About Cashews

Cashews are an excellent substitution for cheese in raw vegan dishes, as they are creamy and smooth in sauces and dressings.

SIMPLE INGREDIENTS

- ½ cup raw cashews, soaked 3-4 hours in water
- ½ cup fresh basil leaves
- 1 fluid ounce fresh-squeezed lemon juice
- 2-3 garlic cloves, minced
- 2 tbsp fresh-squeezed lemon juice
- 1 tsp sea salt
- ¼ cup organic extra virgin olive oil

SIMPLE STEPS

1. Place all ingredients except organic extra virgin olive oil into food processor
2. Puree.
3. Add olive oil little by little until smooth.
4. Taste and add extra garlic, lemon juice, or basil leaves to create a taste that's right for you.

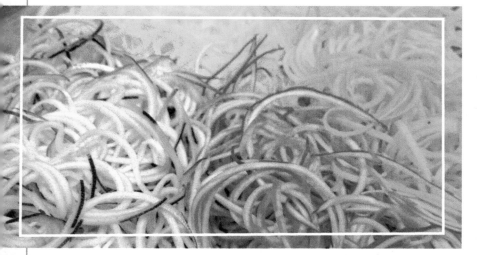

" A raw spiral veggie salad is a perfect way to introduce raw food to everyone, from young kids to adults. It's simple, delicious, and fun to prepare. "

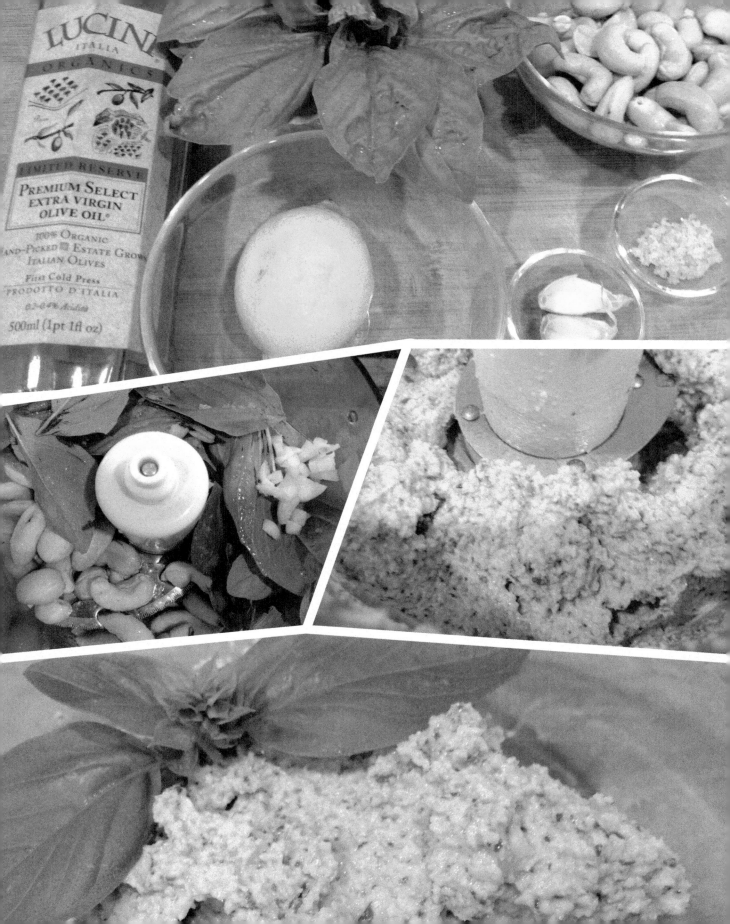

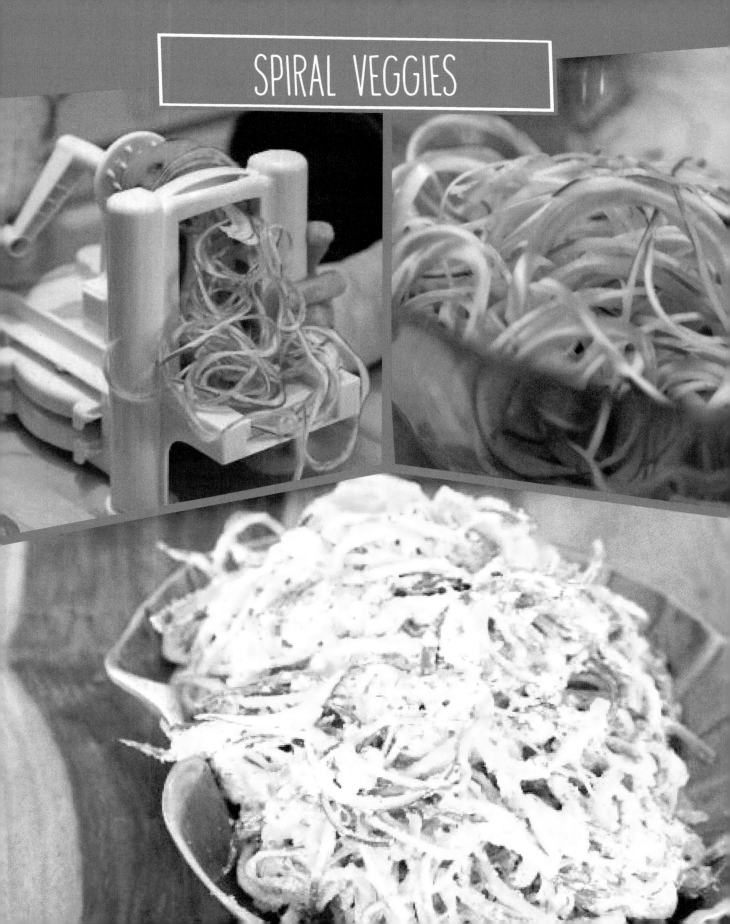

SPIRAL VEGGIES

SIMPLE INGREDIENTS

- 1 large zucchini
- 1 butternut squash, solid end, peeled
- 1 sweet potato
- 1 red beet
- 1 golden beet

SIMPLE STEPS

1. Spiralize veggies into long, pasta-like shapes using a spiral vegetable slicer with a small blade. Be sure to spiralize the red beets last and separate them from the other vegetables to limit bleeding.
2. After spiralizing each vegetable, slice to make the pieces shorter.
3. Allow the vegetables to sit at room temperature to dry.
4. Toss all spiralized vegetables together.
5. Add pesto to the vegetables and toss.
6. Serve and enjoy this fresh raw salad.

" Spiralizing veggies is very mindful and meditative. I love creating the long, beautiful spirals with a rainbow of different-colored vegetables. **"**

Create Your Own Cashew Pesto Dressing

After you've learned the simple cashew pesto technique, create your own flavorful pesto for spiraled vegetables. Experiment with different fresh herbs (parsley, cilantro, or dill), acids (lime juice instead of lemon juice), with or without garlic.

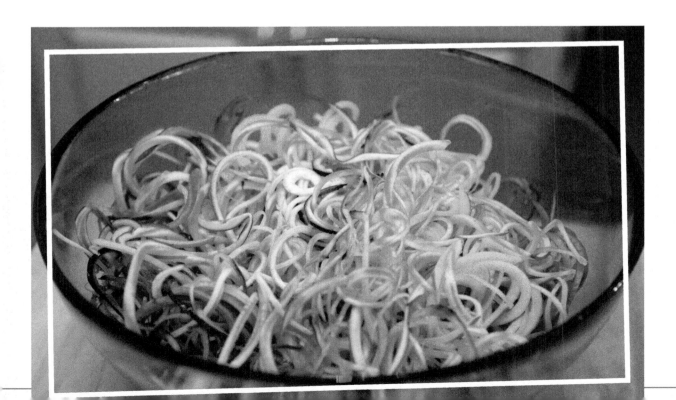

EXPERIENCE NUTRITION™ SIGNATURE AVOCADO SALSA

Honestly, I had never eaten fresh avocados until a few years ago, and thought I didn't like them. One of my brothers made a simple, fresh avocado salsa with his home-grown yellow pear tomatoes and fresh garlic. Since that day when I first experienced the deliciousness of creamy avocados, I loved them and have taught the simple avocado salsa recipe to hundreds of people, including kids, MDs, former NFL players, and holistic students at speaking engagements, workshops, and cooking classes.

Basic Avocado Salsa

Have fun intuitively creating your own avocado salsa with the veggies available right in your own refrigerator.

This simple-to-make avocado salsa (or guacamole) is the best. Make it for lunch, as a snack, or for tailgating parties. It's so easy to prepare and it's so delicious that you'll want to eat it a few times a week. With good monounsaturated fats, fresh veggies, and a squeeze of lemon, enjoy your avocado salsa with your favorite crunchy fresh organic raw veggies.

SIMPLE INGREDIENTS

- 4 soft, ripe avocados
- 2-3 heirloom tomatoes or 6-8 cherry tomatoes
- 3-5 green onions
- Handful fresh cilantro or basil
- 2-3 cloves raw garlic, minced
- Fresh squeezed lemon juice, to taste
- Sea salt to taste

66 Keep an avocado in your kitchen all the time so you're always ready to make a quick avocado salsa to enjoy as a salad or in a wrap. 99

SIMPLE STEPS

1. Chop and gently mix all ingredients.
2. Enjoy as a salad or in a wrap.

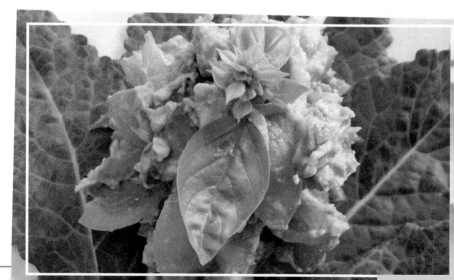

Create Your Own Avocado Salsa

Using the Basic Avocado Salsa Recipe as a guide, create your own with your favorite farmers' market fresh vegetables. Experiment with carrots (orange, yellow, or purple), peppers (red, green, yellow, or purple), cucumbers (green, lemon cucumbers, or Armenian), olives, garbanzo beans, and dehydrated tomatoes.

7 Simple Ways to Enjoy Avocados

1. Homemade avocado salsa
2. Fresh avocado wrap
3. In sandwiches instead of butter or mayonnaise
4. Sliced and added to salad
5. With steamed vegetables
6. In raw vegan desserts
7. With fresh lemon or lime juice, a little sea salt, and minced garlic as a simple snack

Appreciate Your Avocado: How to Grow an Avocado Tree

My parents started an avocado plant in their kitchen and eight years later they were enjoying avocados from their tree. It was amazing to watch the growth process, from a seed, to a small plant, to a tall tree with avocados.

More about avocados

Avocados are primarily monounsaturated fat, which is good for the heart, reduces bad cholesterol, and speeds metabolism. Avocados are a nutritional powerhouse, rich in fiber, potassium, Vitamin C, Vitamin K, folate, and B6.ginger to your food is to use it in a salad dressing.

How to Select the Best Avocado

- Avocados do not ripen on trees; they are harvested when they are deep green and they arrive green at stores.

- Look at the color of the avocado. If it is green, it's not very ripe. If it's darker and blackish, it's riper. To buy the perfect avocado, find one that's a little soft.

- To speed up ripening, place an avocado in a brown bag with an apple or a banana. Check the ripeness for the next two or three days. An avocado is ready to eat when it's black and soft.

- When an avocado reaches its soft black stage, store it in the refrigerator to slow down ripening. Eat it within the next day or two.

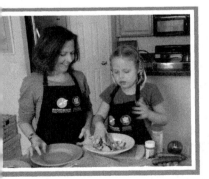

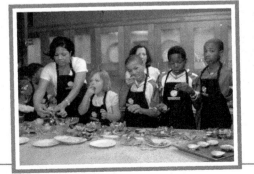

> " I learned to make my own avocado salsa when I was 6 years old. I'm now 11 and make it all the time.
> - **Meredith Albert** "

> " It was fun to have my hands in the avocado.
> - **Kwincy Lassiter** "

Simple Steps to Grow an Avocado Tree

1

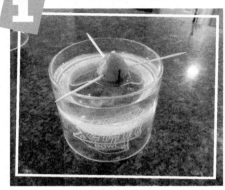

Place an avocado seed in a cup of water with three toothpicks. Be sure the pointy end is up.

2

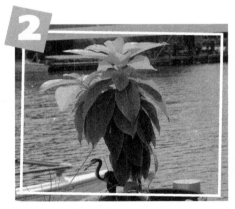

Once the avocado plant has grown to about a foot tall, plant it in soil in a pot.

3

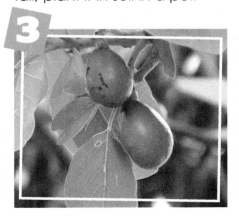

When the tree is a few feet tall, transplant it outside.

SUMMERTIME TOMATO GAZPACHO COLD SOUP

A fresh, cold tomato gazpacho is refreshing, especially on warm days. Make this quick cold tomato soup with red, orange, and yellow tomatoes and red, orange, yellow, and green bell peppers for a bright summer side dish. Be sure to try the beautiful (some may think ugly) heirloom tomatoes. If you are fortunate enough to purchase a whole flat of really ripe organic tomatoes, make a big batch of tomato gazpacho for a summertime picnic.

SIMPLE INGREDIENTS: SOUP

- 10 medium tomatoes, cut into eighths
- 4 red, orange, yellow, and/or green bell peppers, seeded and rough chopped
- 3 cucumbers, rough chopped
- 2 jalapeno or Anaheim peppers, seeded and rough chopped
- ½ cup fresh cilantro, chopped
- ½ cup fresh lime juice
- 6-8 garlic cloves, minced
- Up to 2 cups water, if needed
- Sea salt and pepper, to taste

SIMPLE INGREDIENTS: TOPPING

- 4 tbsp cucumber, small diced
- 4 tbsp tomato, small diced
- 4 tsp cilantro leaves

SIMPLE STEPS

1. Place all soup ingredients in a large bowl.
2. Mix well.
3. Puree half of the ingredients in a high-speed blender until smooth.
4. Combine pureed soup with chopped veggies
5. Taste and season with sea salt and/or pepper.
6. Top with diced cucumbers, tomatoes, and cilantro.
7. Enjoy!
8. Refrigerate leftover gazpacho soup and enjoy the next day for an even more flavorful soup.

Create Your Own Tomato Gazpacho

Use your intuition when you create your tomato gazpacho. Use different colors and types of tomatoes. Sometimes make it chunky; other times make it smooth. Try different levels of spiciness using jalapeno or Anaheim peppers. Sometimes make it spicy hot, sometimes make it mild. Try different types of in-season cucumbers, such Armenian, pickling, or lemon.

> " The key to a beautiful tomato gazpacho is to blend some of the fresh veggies into a creamy liquid and to keep some veggies chunky. "

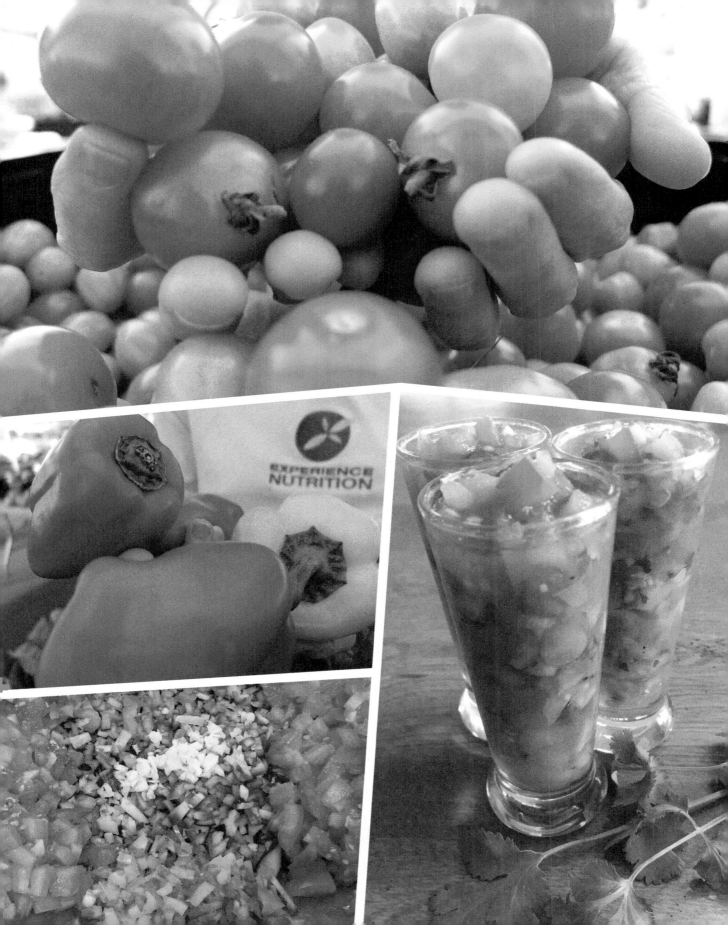

KALE CHIPS: DEHYDRATED AND BAKED

Kale is such a popular food, eaten as a salad, chips, or a wrap. Here's a very quick way to make delicious dehydrated kale chips. Once you have learned to make dehydrated kale chips, you can easily change the flavor with different spices and herbs, such as fresh ginger, basil, or oregano.

SIMPLE INGREDIENTS

- 2 large bunches kale, dinosaur or curly green, torn into pieces
- 1 cup raw cashews, pre-soaked in water 4-6 hours
- 1 fresh lemon, approximately 2 tbsp lemon juice
- ¼ cup nutritional yeast
- 2 tsp onion powder
- 1 tsp garlic powder
- ¼ tsp sea salt
- ½-⅔ cup water

SIMPLE STEPS

1. Soak cashews for 4-6 hours in water. Once soft, drain.
2. Wash kale, remove the leaves from the stems, and tear leaves into big pieces.
3. Place lemon juice, nutritional yeast, onion powder, and garlic powder into high-speed blender.
4. Add about half of the water and blend.
5. Continue to add more water, if needed, to create a thick, pourable dressing.
6. To prepare the kale chips, place the kale pieces into a large bowl and pour dressing over the kale.
7. Using your hands, thoroughly coat the kale leaves with the dressing.
8. Place the kale leaves onto dehydrator trays, making sure that the leaves are in a single layer so that they dehydrate evenly.
9. Dehydrate at 115°F for approximately 7 hours or until dehydrated and crisp.

SIMPLE STEPS TO BAKE KALE CHIPS

1. Preheat oven to 275°F.
2. Line 2 large, flat baking sheets with parchment paper.
3. Place kale leaves on the baking sheet in a single layer.
4. Bake for 40-45 minutes, turning leaves halfway through cooking.

Kale leaves

Keep kale leaves as large as possible, as they will shrink when dehydrated or baked in the oven.

Nutritional yeast

Nutritional yeast, a fungus grown on molasses, is a complete protein, rich in vitamin B12. It melts and has a mild Cheddar cheese flavor, and adds flavor to kale chips, sauces, and soups.

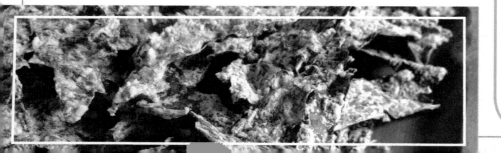

What is Dehydrating?

Dehydrating is the process of removing the moisture from food by surrounding food with a warm circulation of air, not exceeding 118 degrees Fahrenheit. This process concentrates flavors and creates dry, crisp food.

Dehydrating is a simple, quick way to prepare food for different types of people and various culinary uses:

- **Raw Diet.** Raw foodists (who eat food that is not cooked above 118 degrees) dehydrate lots of fruit, vegetables, wraps, and crackers with nuts and seeds for everyday eating.

- **Simple Fruit.** Kids and adults of all ages enjoy dehydrated fruit (bananas, apples, persimmons) for everyday snacks.

- **Culinary Delight.** Chefs and culinary enthusiasts dehydrate to concentrate and intensify the flavor of food, such as tomatoes, sweet peppers, and beets.

How to Shop for a High-Quality Dehydrator

A dehydrator, sometimes referred to as a "raw oven," is an essential tool for the raw kitchen. When shopping for a dehydrator, look for one with the heating unit in the back, as it creates a constant circulation of air in the box, which allows for the evaporation of moisture from the food. Through the removal of moisture, the foods are properly preserved without spoilage and harmful bacterial growth. Excalibur and Sedona are two popular brands. Teflex sheets (or parchment paper) are used to dehydrate foods, such as fruit or vegetables, with higher moisture content.

Round Dehydrators

Round dehydrators with fans on the top or bottom do not dry food as evenly and require manual shifting of the trays to optimize drying consistency.

" If you invest in a dehydrator, I recommend one with a timer and multiple heating temperatures for consistency and ease in preparing raw foods. "

Action: No Recipe Fun!

Now that you have experimented with salads, cold soup, kale chips, and avocado salsa, look in your refrigerator and be creative, using your intuition to create your own salad, soup, or salsa.

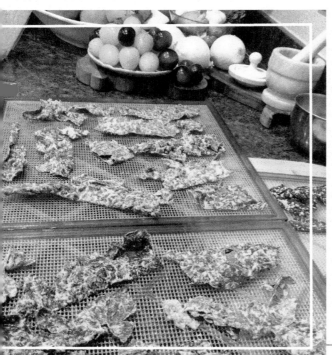

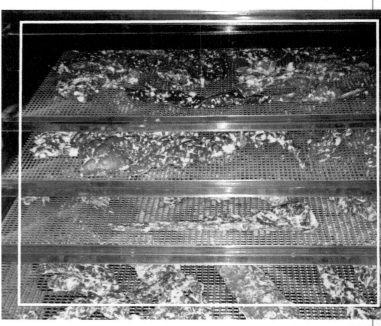

Create Soups, Sauces & Pestos with Everyday Veggies

Culinary

- Mindfully chop veggies and make veggie stock
- Cook stock and use it later
- How to quickly steam veggies in a bamboo steamer
- How to stovetop pan-fry fresh herbs for garnishing
- Create a variety of tomato sauces
- How and why to sweat onions
- Simple steps to dehydrate tomatoes
- Use a serrated tomato knife
- Simple avocado dressing
- Simple steps to roast peppers

Recipes

- Basic Organic Veggie Stock
- Vegan Dairy-free Butternut Squash Soup
- Simple Stovetop Sauteed Tomato Sauce
- Simple Roasted Tomatoes Sauce
- Raw Tomatoes with Salads and Avocados
- Vegan Dairy-free Roasted Pepper Pesto
- Olives and Sun-dried Tomato Tapenade

Nutrition

- Eat cooked tomatoes

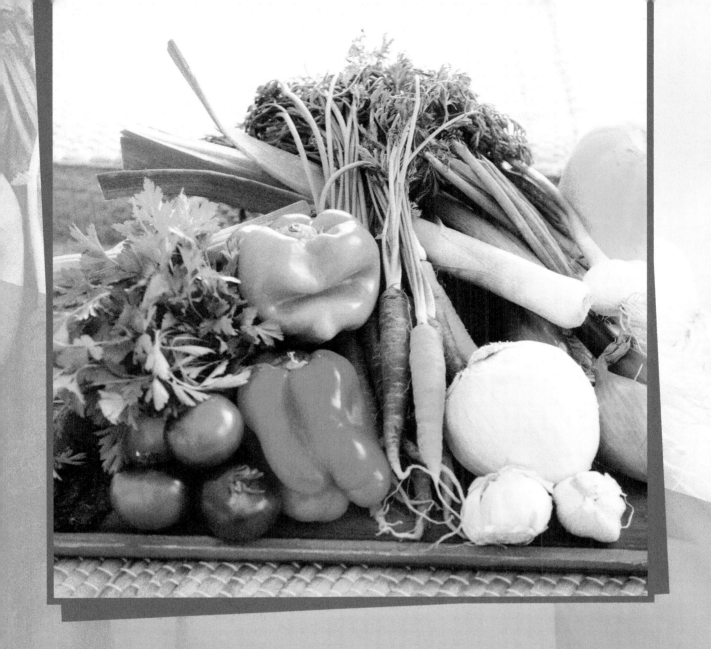

CREATE SOUPS, SAUCES AND PESTOS WITH
EVERYDAY VEGGIES

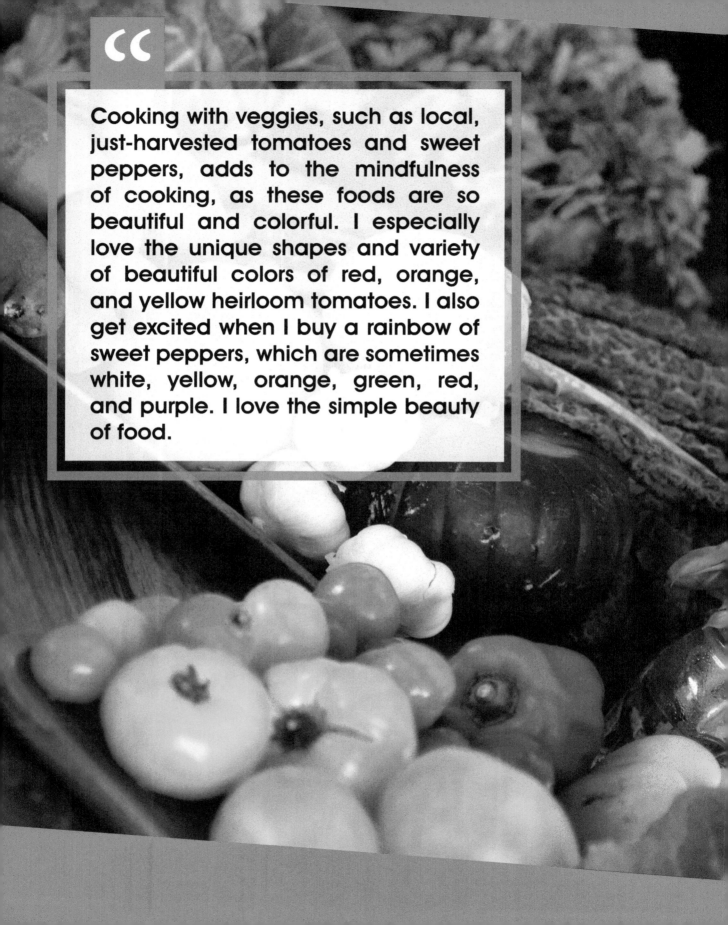

Cooking with veggies, such as local, just-harvested tomatoes and sweet peppers, adds to the mindfulness of cooking, as these foods are so beautiful and colorful. I especially love the unique shapes and variety of beautiful colors of red, orange, and yellow heirloom tomatoes. I also get excited when I buy a rainbow of sweet peppers, which are sometimes white, yellow, orange, green, red, and purple. I love the simple beauty of food.

CREATE SOUPS, SAUCES AND PESTOS WITH EVERYDAY VEGGIES

Cooking simple soups, tomato sauce, and pestos is fun

Often, people eat soup, tomato sauce, or pesto only from a can or jar. Now is the time to enjoy making your own. Creating veggie stock and soup is a very mindful, meditative process, and full of natural food aromatherapy in the kitchen. Experimenting with tomatoes, especially in-season and locally grown, invites natural creativity and intuitive cooking. Pestos with roasted peppers and sun-dried tomatoes showcase the intense, vibrant flavors of these veggies.

In this section you will learn how to:

- Mindfully chop organic veggies and make your own veggie stock.
- Create a smooth, vegan, dairy-free butternut squash soup.
- Quickly steam veggies in a bamboo steamer.
- Stovetop fry fresh herbs for soup garnish.
- Create a variety of simple sauces with fresh in-season tomatoes.
- Sweat an onion as a sweet base for culinary creations.
- Roast peppers for pesto.
- Create a vegan, dairy-free roasted pepper pesto.
- Create a gourmet-quality olive and sun-dried tomato tapenade.

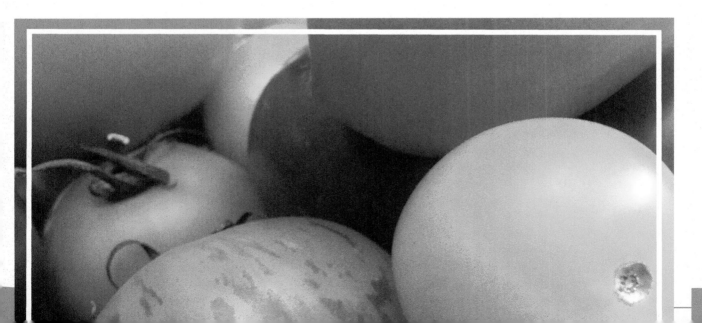

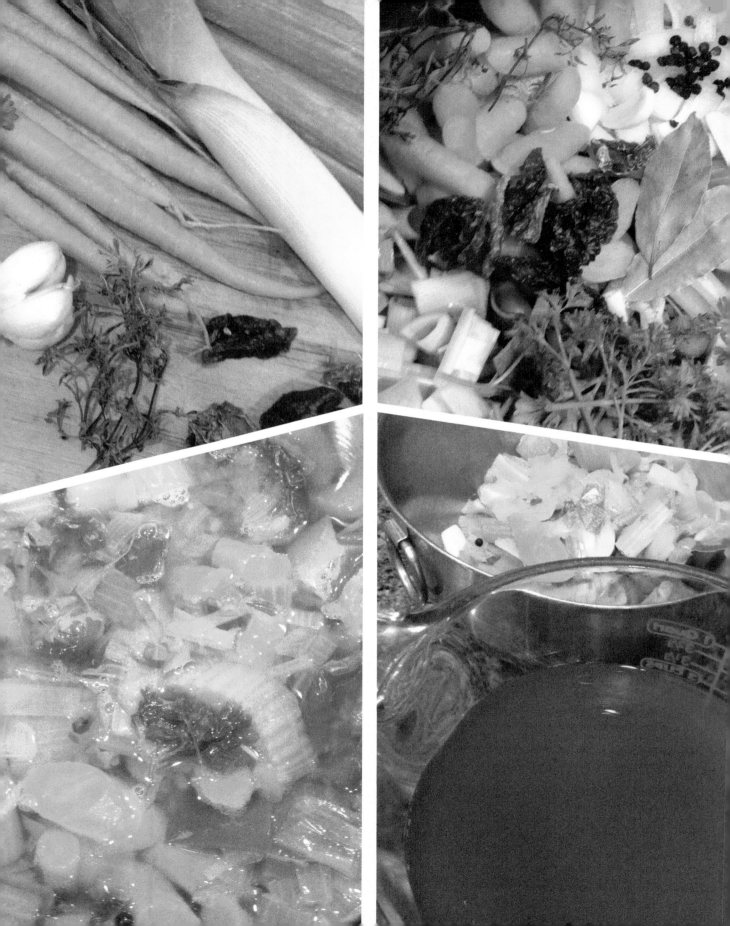

BASIC ORGANIC VEGGIE STOCK

Make your own veggie stock and enjoy the mindfulness of chopping veggies, the beauty of all the ingredients in the stock, and the natural aromatherapy of simmering stock. Be proud that you have made stock to use as a base for other culinary creations. Use your veggie stock as the foundation for soups and sauces, add it to quinoa for rich flavor, and use it to sauté veggies.

Basic Veggie Stock: Start with High-Quality Organic Ingredients

Deep, flavorful stock adds depth and richness to other dishes. Because stock is a base for other culinary creations, including soup, sauces, and sautés, it's important to start the foundation – the stock – with high-quality organic ingredients.

SIMPLE INGREDIENTS

- 4 carrots, chopped
- ½ head celery, chopped
- 2 large onions, chopped
- 1 leek, white and green parts, chopped
- 3-6 garlic cloves, peeled
- 1 tsp black peppercorns
- 2 bay leaves
- ¼ cup sun-dried tomatoes
- ¼ cup fresh parsley, chopped
- Few sprigs thyme
- 8 cups cold water

SIMPLE STEPS

1. Cook the stock.
   - Roughly chop all vegetables
   - Place all fresh ingredients in a large (6- to 8-quart) stock pot.
   - Add water.
   - Bring to a boil.
   - Lower heat to simmer.
   - Simmer, uncovered, for 1-1½ hours.
   - Allow stock to cool for 15-20 minutes.
2. Strain the stock with cheesecloth or a food mill.
   - Line a strainer with cheesecloth and place it on top of a large bowl.
   - Pour stock into the strainer, allowing the liquid to pour through.
   - Squeeze veggies with the cheesecloth to release all liquid.

Tip for stock

If you'd like to use some of the stock later, freeze 1-cup servings in a plastic bag or container. When you're ready to use the stock, defrost it in a bowl of cold water.

" I love the mindfulness of chopping veggies for soup stock, and every time I make stock I enjoy the sweet, natural aromatherapy of the simmering veggies. The simmering stock brings back warm memories of my childhood, when our whole house smelled like celery and onions when my mom cooked homemade soup. "

VEGAN DAIRY-FREE BUTTERNUT SQUASH SOUP

Create your own easy-to-prepare sweet, creamy butternut squash soup. Garnish with pan-fried herbs and a drizzle of oil (walnut, pumpkin seed, or olive oil) for a beautiful presentation. When served warm in the fall, butternut squash soup is ideal for a chilly Thanksgiving. Served cold in the summer, it's perfect for a picnic.

SIMPLE INGREDIENTS

- 1 ½ tbsp organic extra virgin olive oil
- 3 shallots, minced
- 2 ½ cups butternut squash, peeled and steamed until fork tender
- 3 ½ cups veggie stock
- 2 tbsp sweetener: maple syrup, molasses, or brown rice syrup
- ¾ tsp sea salt
- 1 tbsp olive, walnut, or pumpkin seed oil
- Pan-fried basil for garnish

SIMPLE STEPS

1. Gather your mise en place.
2. To prepare the soup, preheat a (6- to 8-quart) soup pot to medium.
3. Add olive oil to the pot.
4. Add shallots and sauté until golden and translucent.
5. Pour steamed butternut squash, veggie stock, sweetener, and sea salt into the pot.
6. Simmer and cook for 10-15 minutes.
7. Using a blender or hand-stick blender, blend until smooth.
8. Garnish with pan-fried basil and a drizzle of olive, walnut, or pumpkin seed oil.

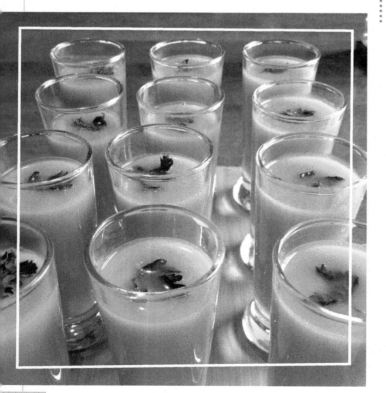

Create Your Own Soup

After you've learned the simple soup cooking process with butternut squash, intuitively create your own soups with different winter squash, such as acorn or pumpkin, or even sweet potatoes. Experiment with various herbs and oils as a garnish.

> " I usually prefer chunky, rustic veggie soup, but once I learned this butternut squash technique to make a smooth, creamy soup, I now enjoy creamy, dairy-free, vegan soups throughout the year. "

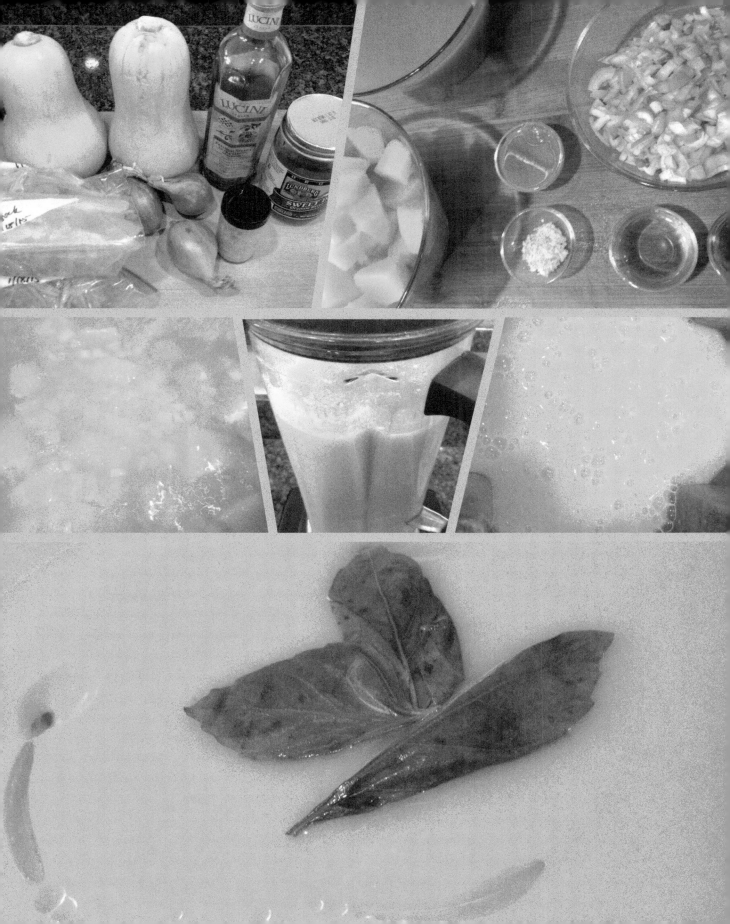

How to Quickly Steam Veggies in a Bamboo Steamer

Using a bamboo steamer to steam veggies is simple, quick, and efficient. Plus, the veggies are nutrient-rich, as the nutrients stay in the vegetables. Experiment with steaming all kinds of farmers' market fresh vegetables, including asparagus, beets, broccoli, cauliflower, carrots, snap peas, and sweet potatoes.

SIMPLE STEPS

1. Fill a large (6- to 8-quart) soup pot with 2-3 inches of water, place over medium-high heat, and bring to boil.
2. Slice veggies into even-sized chunks.
3. Place vegetables in bamboo steamer baskets, being mindful that the veggies are not touching each other to allow the steam from the boiling water to cook them. Place denser food (like roots) on the bottom basket and lighter vegetables on the top.
4. Sprinkle veggies with a little sea salt.
5. Place bamboo steamer over the boiling water.
6. Cover with lid.
7. Steam for about 5 minutes or until just cooked.
8. After the veggies have cooked, use them in your recipe.

How to Pan-Fry Herbs for Garnishing

Basil and parsley are beautiful, crispy garnish. Use neutral-tasting grapeseed oil to quickly fry the herbs, since it does not add flavor to them.

SIMPLE INGREDIENTS

- ½ cup grapeseed oil
- ½ cup fresh basil or parsley leaves

SIMPLE STEPS

1. Cut herb leaves into small pieces and place on paper towel to air dry.
2. Place grapeseed oil into a small fry pan and heat over medium.
3. When the oil is slightly bubbling, using a slotted spoon, lower the herbs into the oil.
4. Fry the herbs for 5-10 seconds, until they become even in color.
5. Transfer to a plate with a paper towel to drain.
6. Use to garnish soup.

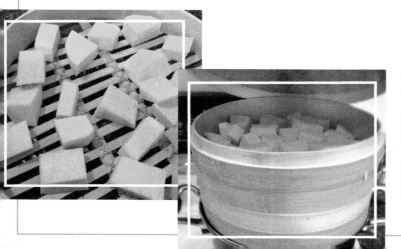

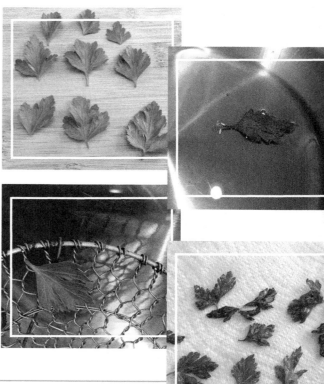

Raw Tomatoes in Salads and with Avocados

A rainbow of raw tomatoes adds freshness and beauty to all salads, including simple avocado spinach salad, created with what's available at the farmers' market.

SIMPLE INGREDIENTS

- Tomatoes, chopped
- Spinach, torn into bite-size pieces
- Cucumber, sliced
- Red pepper, sliced
- Avocado
- Fresh lime juice
- Fresh parsley
- Sea salt

SIMPLE STEPS

1. Gather your mise en place.
2. Gently massage the spinach with avocado, lime juice, and sea salt.
3. Toss in the red pepper, tomatoes, and cucumber.
4. Plate and enjoy!

How and Why We Sweat Onions

Sweating is the gentlest dry-heat cooking method. Sweating, a "low and slow" technique, is often the first step to developing flavor in a dish. Vegetables that are sweat form the first layer of flavor in a dish. Finely cut vegetables (such as onions, leeks, celery, and carrots) are coated in fat and cooked very slowly over very low heat until completely softened. The goal is to slowly release the flavor of the vegetables without browning them. Sweating is used to create a base for soups, tomato sauce, and dishes with a light color, where caramelized vegetables would change the appearance of a dish.

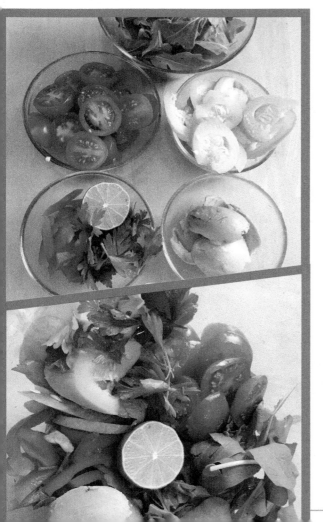

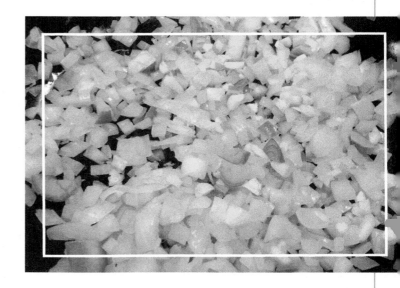

Simple Avocado Dressing

The simple rule to make a salad dressing is to use a fat, an acid, and sea salt. The dressing for this simple tomato salad features avocado as the fat, lime as the acid, and the sea salt.

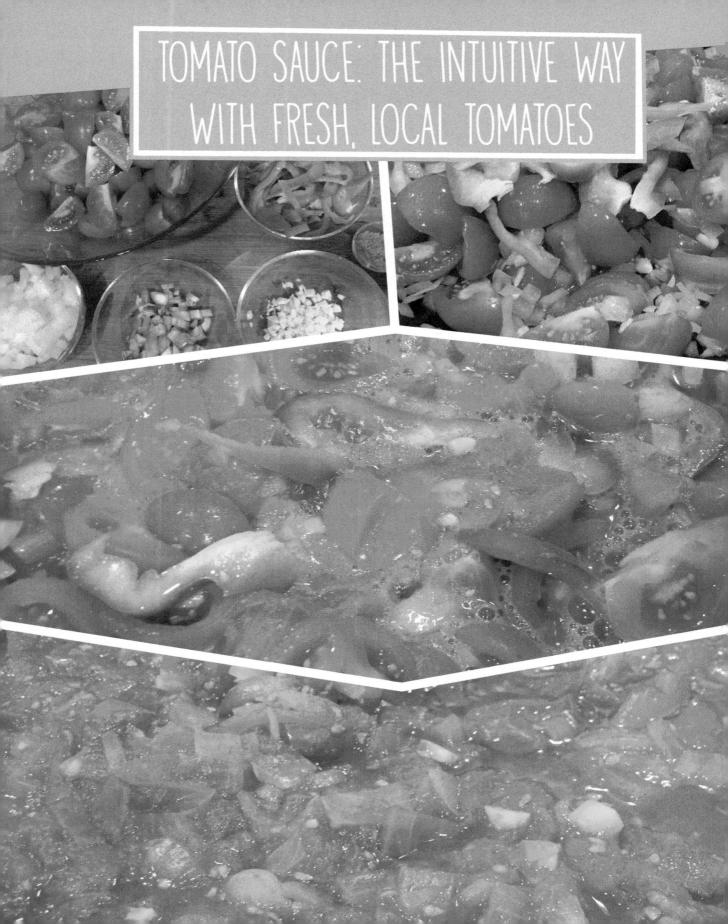

TOMATO SAUCE: THE INTUITIVE WAY WITH FRESH, LOCAL TOMATOES

A few times a year, I have the opportunity to purchase a whole flat of really ripe locally grown Arizona organic tomatoes that must be cooked in a day or two. One of our local Arizona farmers sells these ripe tomatoes at an incredible price of $15 for 20 pounds. Of course, I purchase them and then intuitively cook tomatoes for a few days.

> " When I see the big flats of overly ripe organic tomatoes available at the farmers' market, I get so excited, I can feel my heart beating faster. I start to intuitively visualize what I'd like to cook, and I buy other staple ingredients, like onions and garlic, that I'll use to cook with the tomatoes. "

Simple Stovetop Sautéed Tomato Sauce

With the focus on the tomatoes, a stovetop tomato sauce is thick and very aromatic with garlic and onions.

SIMPLE INGREDIENTS

- 5-6 cups tomatoes, chopped in quarters
- 1 tbsp organic extra virgin olive oil
- 1 red onion, diced
- 1 shallot, minced
- 5-7 cloves fresh garlic, minced
- 2-3 green peppers, sliced
- Sea salt

SIMPLE STEPS

1. Gather your mise en place.
2. Place olive oil and onion in a large sauté pan.
3. Turn heat on low and sweat the onion with the olive oil for about 6-7 minutes, until the onion is translucent.
4. Add the shallot and sweat with the onion for another 5 minutes.
5. Add tomatoes, green pepper, and salt to the sauté pan.
6. Increase heat to medium.
7. Simmer for about an hour, stirring occasionally.
8. Enjoy with roasted spaghetti squash or freeze to use later.

Eat Cooked Tomatoes

Tomatoes are delicious when ripe; however, to get the most nutritional value out of them, cook tomatoes with a little fat. Lycopene is a powerful antioxidant in tomatoes and has demonstrated a protective role in heart disease and cancers, including prostate, colon, and rectal. Lycopene in tomatoes is more available for the body when it comes from cooked tomatoes than when it comes from raw ones. Since lycopene is fat soluble, cook tomatoes with some fat, such as organic olive oil, to help facilitate the absorption of lycopene into the body.

How to Freeze Tomato Sauce

If you will not use all of your tomato sauce within a few days, freeze it in plastic bags or containers and use it within six months. When you're ready to use the sauce with sautéed veggies or roasted spaghetti sauce, place the sauce in a sauce pan with a little water over medium-low heat, and occasionally stir until it is defrosted and ready to use in your cooking.

Simple Roasted Tomatoes Sauce

Oven-roasted tomato sauce is very easy to cook. The main ingredient is time. Be creative with the quantity and combination of tomatoes, onions, carrot, and garlic when you roast this beautiful, delicious sauce. Use the sauce with veggies or, to make soup, strain the cooked tomatoes through cheesecloth, then blend into a creamy soup.

SIMPLE INGREDIENTS

- Tomatoes
- Red onion, sliced
- Few carrots, chopped
- Few garlic cloves, sliced
- Sea salt

SIMPLE STEPS

1. Place whole tomatoes in a large roasting pan.
2. Add the onions, carrots, garlic, and sea salt and lightly toss.
3. Roast at 350 degrees for about 3 hours, stirring every 45 minutes.
4. Enjoy the aroma of the roasting tomatoes.

Serrated Tomato Knife

To easily cut tomatoes, use a small serrated knife with an up-and-down cutting motion. Years ago I did not at all enjoy cutting tomatoes, but now with my little 5-inch serrated knife, I cut them quickly and smoothly, without the juice of the tomato squirting out.

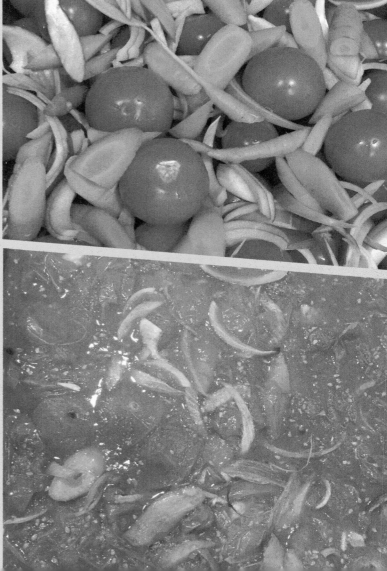

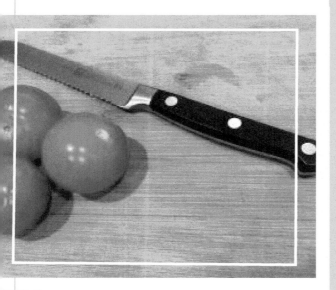

Simple Steps to Dehydrate Tomatoes

Dehydrating tomatoes is very simple. Dehydrating concentrates flavor and creates intensely sweet tomatoes. Use dehydrated tomatoes to accent dishes such as avocado salsa, salads, stir-fries, and hummus, or even eat them as a sweet snack.

SIMPLE INGREDIENTS

• Tomatoes

SIMPLE STEPS

1. Cut tomatoes into ¼-inch slices.
2. Place tomatoes flat on dehydrator sheets so that they're not touching.
3. Dehydrate at 125 degrees for 5-9 hours.
4. Enjoy the deep, intense sweetness of the tomatoes with soups, salad, avocados, pesto, or even as a snack.

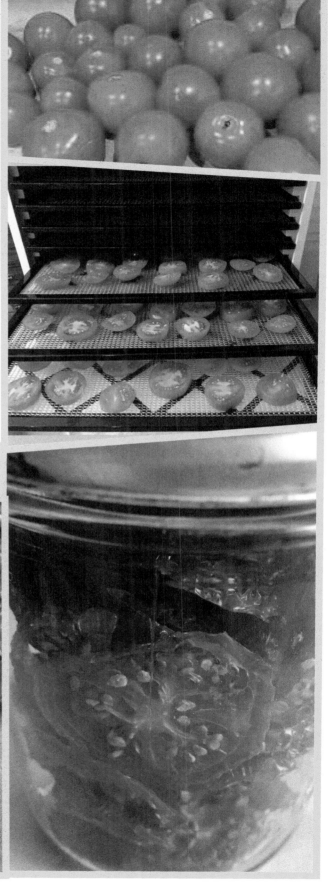

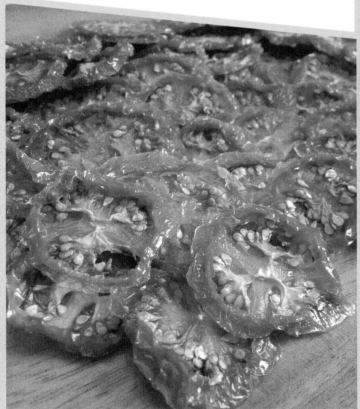

VEGAN DAIRY-FREE ROASTED PEPPER PESTO

Homemade pestos add extra interest to wraps, salads, raw vegetables, and crackers. This simple pesto pairs well with cucumbers for a light appetizer.

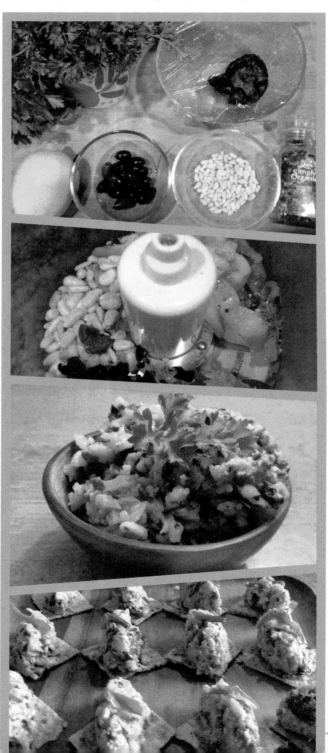

SIMPLE INGREDIENTS

- 2 cups roasted peppers
- 1/3 cup pine nuts, toasted
- 2 tbsp lemon zest
- 1/4 cup Kalamata olives, chopped
- 2 tbsp fresh herb (parsley or basil)

SIMPLE STEPS

1. Place all ingredients, except the fresh herb in a food processor.
2. Pulse until mixture is coarsely chopped.
3. Add the fresh herb and pulse to blend.
4. Enjoy with cucumbers or a raw cracker.

Simple Steps to Roast Peppers

Roasted blackened peppers add earthy richness to pestos and hummus.

SIMPLE INGREDIENTS

- 5-6 large red, orange, or yellow peppers

SIMPLE STEPS

1. Preheat broiler to high.
2. Place peppers on a foil-lined baking sheet.
3. Broil each side of the peppers until blistered and blackened. Turn to blacken each side.
4. Place peppers in a bowl, cover with plastic wrap, and let sit for 10 minutes. The peppers will sweat and skins will loosen.
5. After peppers are cool, place a strainer over a bowl and peel the skin from the peppers while the liquid drains into the bowl.
6. Use the peppers in a pesto or hummus.

Olives and Sun-Dried Tomato Tapenade

Sun-dried tomato and olive spread is a tasty topping for farmers' market fresh raw veggies.

SIMPLE INGREDIENTS

- 1-2 cloves garlic
- 1 ½ cups Kalamata olives, pitted
- ½ cup sun-dried tomatoes
- 2 tbsp capers
- 2 tbsp fresh parsley
- $^1/_3$-½ cup olive oil

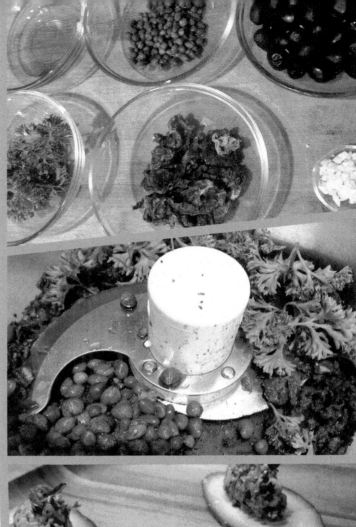

SIMPLE STEPS

1. Gather your mise en place.
2. Roughly chop the sun-dried tomatoes; drain oil, if needed.
3. In a food processor, mince garlic.
4. Add olives and pulse until fine, not paste-like.
5. Remove olive and garlic mixture from the food processor.
6. Place sun-dried tomatoes in food processor and blend until fine.
7. Add capers and parsley and pulse a few times.
8. Mix olive/garlic mixture with sun-dried tomatoes/capers/parsley mixture by hand.
9. Add olive oil until you reach desired consistency.
10. Enjoy the pesto on veggies or raw crackers.

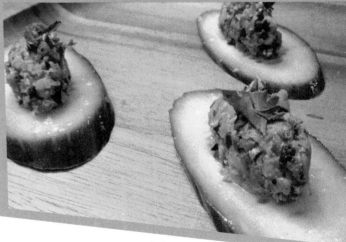

Action: Experiment with Tomatoes and try a pesto or tapenade

In this section, we have created different dishes with tomatoes. I invite you to experiment with a batch of tomatoes and cook a few sauces, enjoy them raw, and, if you have a dehydrator, dehydrate a batch for garnish or as a flavorful sweet snack. Also, create a pesto or tapenade for a delicious appetizer or snack.

" I learned how to make simple, fresh pestos during my professional plant-based culinary certification. Once I learned how simple it is to prepare pestos with a few interesting, impactful, flavorful ingredients, such as a roasted pepper or sun-dried tomatoes, I now create pestos with different types of nuts and herbs. "

Simple Ways to Cook Amazing Roots

Culinary
- Quickly steam carrots in a bamboo steamer
- Finish carrots with fresh cumin seeds and lemon dressing
- Roast all kinds of roots
- 7 culinary tips for great roasted roots
- 5 ways to finish roasted roots
- Be creative with beets in a bag
- Slow roast golden beets in parchment paper bag
- Make dairy-free raw cashew cream
- Steps to bake sweet potatoes
- Bake sweet potato and chickpea burgers
- What's the Difference: Sauté vs. Stir-fry

Recipes
- Bamboo Steamer Carrots with Cumin Seed Lemon Dressing
- Sweet & Rich Roasted Roots
- Slow Roasted Golden Beets in a Parchment Paper Bag
- Raw Cashew Cream
- Sweet Potato & Chickpea Burgers
- Simple Veggie Stir-Fry with Roots and In-Season Produce

Nutrition
- Why roots are good for us

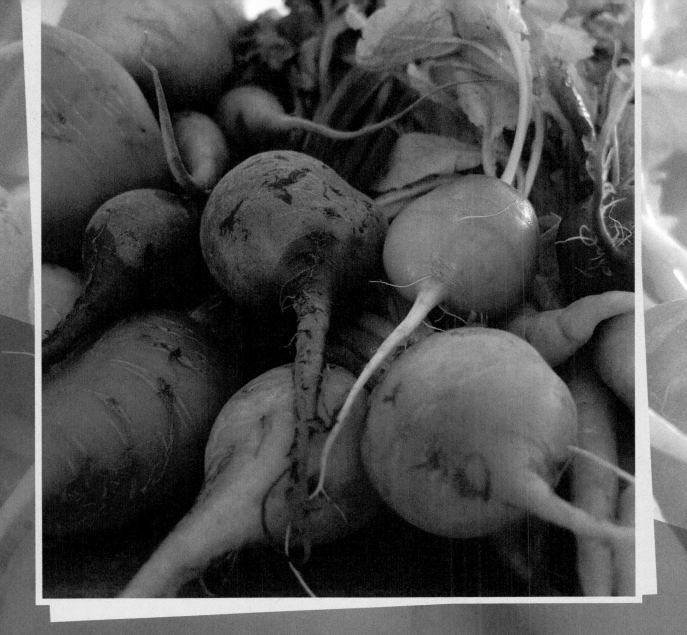

SIMPLE WAYS TO COOK
AMAZING ROOTS

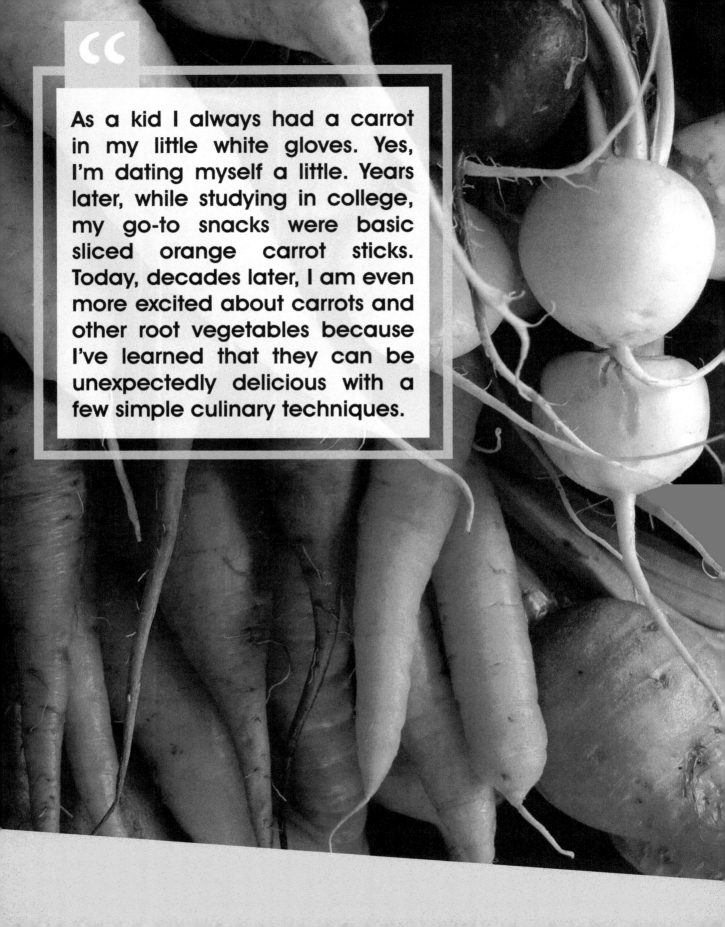

As a kid I always had a carrot in my little white gloves. Yes, I'm dating myself a little. Years later, while studying in college, my go-to snacks were basic sliced orange carrot sticks. Today, decades later, I am even more excited about carrots and other root vegetables because I've learned that they can be unexpectedly delicious with a few simple culinary techniques.

SIMPLE WAYS TO COOK AMAZING ROOTS

Root vegetables of all kinds are so naturally sweet when cooked, mindfully beautiful, and delicious

The key to enjoying roots is to know how to cook them with simple techniques that bring out their naturally sweet, sometimes earthy flavor. All you need are a few basic culinary methods such as roasting, stir-frying, and steaming, as well as finishing with a light dressing. Plus, you can make veggie burgers with sweet potatoes. Once you learn these simple techniques, you can creatively and intuitively experiment and cook with all kinds of beautiful, local, in-season, farmers' market vegetables for meals or side dishes.

In this section you will learn how to:

- Quickly steam carrots in a bamboo steamer to bring out their natural flavor.
- Finish carrots with a simple fresh cumin seed lemon dressing.
- Roast all kinds of roots on natural parchment paper to create perfect veggies with a crisp, caramelized exterior and soft, moist interior.
- Slow roast golden beets with herbs in parchment paper for a gourmet side dish.
- Make dairy-free raw cashew cream.
- Bake sweet potato and chickpea burgers to eat as a snack any time.
- Create a simple veggie stir-fry with roots and in-season produce.

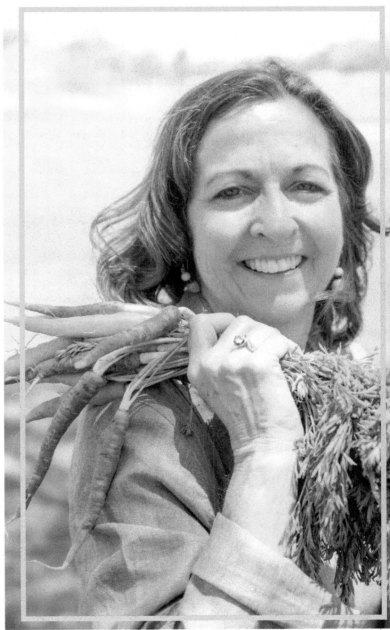

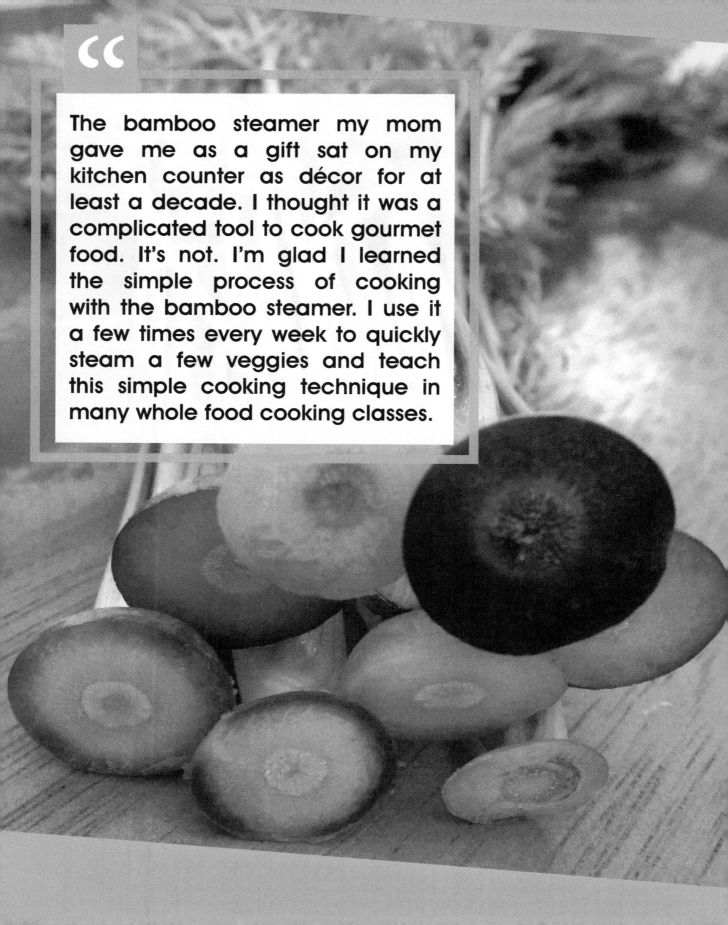

The bamboo steamer my mom gave me as a gift sat on my kitchen counter as décor for at least a decade. I thought it was a complicated tool to cook gourmet food. It's not. I'm glad I learned the simple process of cooking with the bamboo steamer. I use it a few times every week to quickly steam a few veggies and teach this simple cooking technique in many whole food cooking classes.

BAMBOO STEAMER CARROTS

A bamboo steamer is key to the new view of the year-round healthy eating kitchen. First, learn to steam carrots with the mindful process of steaming. Once you learn how to steam carrots, use your bamboo steamer to steam all kinds of veggies.Try a rustic medley of roots such as carrots, sweet potatoes, and golden beets. Or quickly cook butternut squash and pumpkin as the base for a warm fall soup. Also, experiment with steaming a mix of spring veggies like asparagus, Brussels sprouts, collard greens, and kale.

Bamboo Steamer Carrots with Cumin Seed Lemon Dressing

Finishing carrots with a simple herb and citrus dressing adds richness to the simple carrot. Enjoy creating a cumin seed lemon dressing by toasting cumin seeds for added flavor and aromatherapy, lightly tossing the carrots by hand with the dressing and mindfully plating your carrots. Enjoy!

SIMPLE INGREDIENTS

- 6-8 large carrots, rainbow if available, sliced
- ½ tsp cumin seeds
- Pinch sea salt
- 2 tbsp flat-leaf parsley
- ½ fresh lemon
- 2-3 tbsp walnut oil (or extra virgin olive oil)

SIMPLE STEPS

1. Steam Carrots
   - To set up the bamboo steamer, fill a large (6- to 8-quart) soup pot with 3-4 inches of water, place over high heat, and bring to a boil.
   - Place sliced carrots into the bamboo steamer. Spread out the carrots so that they do not touch each other to allow the steam to rise and cook the carrots. Sprinkle carrots with a pinch of sea salt.
   - Place bamboo steamer on top of the pot with steaming water. Cover with lid and let steam for about 5-7 minutes or until just cooked.
   - Test the carrots for doneness. When carrots easily come off a fork, they're ready.
   - Once the carrots have finished cooking, pour them into a large bowl.
2. Cumin Seed Lemon Finishing Dressing
   - While the carrots are steaming, prepare the finishing dressing.
   - To toast the cumin seeds, heat a small sauté pan over low heat. Add the seeds to the pan and cook lightly until fragrant. Once done, remove the seeds from the pan.
   - To make the dressing, gather the lemon and oil, and roughly chop the parsley.
   - Squeeze the lemon juice on the carrots and drizzle with the oil. Gently toss with your hands to coat. Add the toasted cumin seeds and sprinkle with a little salt. Add the parsley and toss again.
   - Mindfully plate and enjoy.

Add Flavor to Steamed Veggies

To add unique, interesting flavors to steamed veggies finish them with oils and fresh herbs. When finishing steamed vegetables, such as carrots, asparagus, broccoli, and Brussels sprouts, experiment with different nut oils (almond, hazelnut, walnut) and different fresh herbs (basil, lemon balm, oregano, parsley). Enjoy using your intuition to create fresh, in-season organic veggies with a variety of tastes.

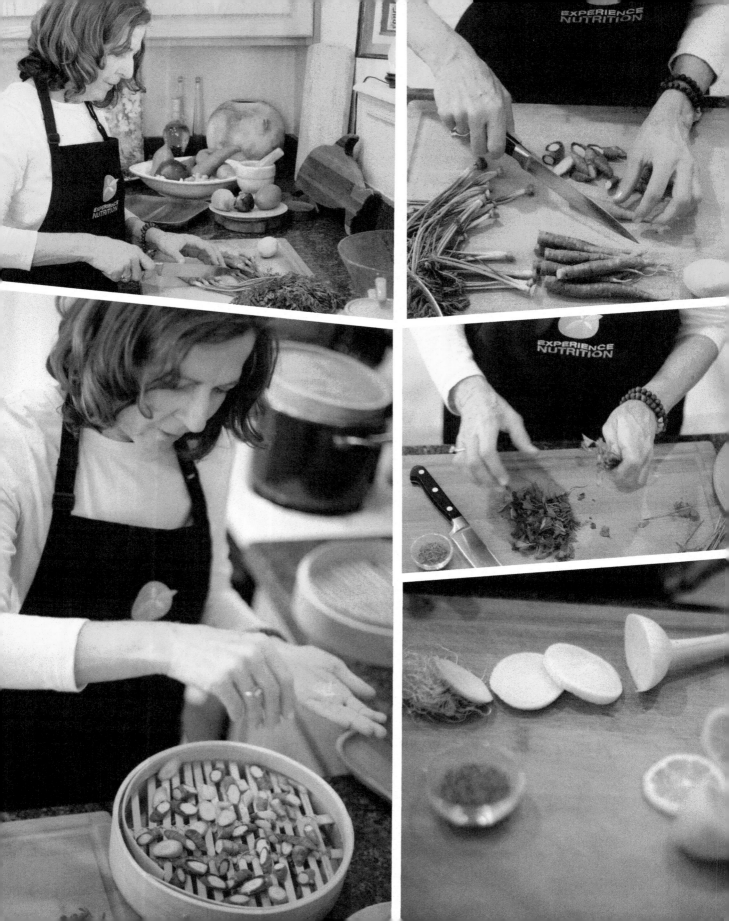

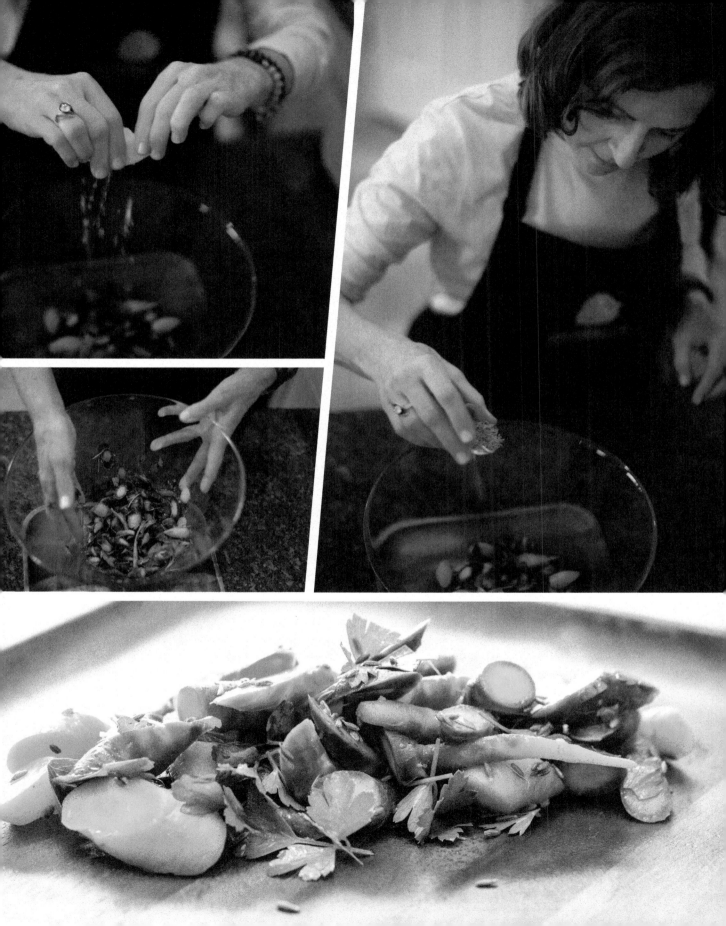

SWEET AND RICH ROASTED ROOTS

Roasted roots are beautiful, flavorful, and sweet, as well as a rich, colorful complement to any meal. The roasting culinary technique is a dry heat cooking method that intensifies and concentrates the flavor of vegetables. When roasted properly, the natural sugars in the vegetables brown or caramelize to create a deep, rich flavor. When visiting your farmers' market, buy a few roots even if you don't recognize them, and roast them with this simple, quick culinary technique. Enjoy roasted roots as a side dish, to create soup, with hummus, or in a raw kale salad or veggie wrap.

SIMPLE INGREDIENTS

- 10-12 of your favorite roots: carrots, sweet potatoes, parsnips, golden beets, red beets, and radishes
- Approximately ¼ cup organic extra virgin olive oil
- 3 tbsp dry herbs (Choose a few: basil, marjoram, oregano, rosemary, sage, or thyme)
- ½ tsp sea salt

SIMPLE STEPS

1. Pre-heat oven to 475 degrees F.
2. Scrub roots under running water to clean the outside.
3. Let sit for about 10 minutes to dry.
4. Slice roots into even, bite-size pieces.
5. Mix olive oil, herbs, and sea salt in a bowl to make the dressing.
6. Add root vegetables to the bowl and toss to evenly coat with the dressing.
7. Carefully lay the roots on parchment paper in a heavy-duty flat baking sheet pan. Place roots flat side down in a single layer, making sure the vegetables do not touch.
8. Place baking sheet on the middle rack of the oven.
9. Roast roots in the oven for about 20 minutes, then turn vegetables.
10. Cook another 15 minutes, until fork tender.
11. Plate vegetables. Finish with a drizzle of olive oil.
12. Enjoy!

> " In my public and private hands-on cooking classes, I encourage participants to experiment with different herbs and spices for roasted roots. A fun way to intuitively choose herbs is to close your eyes, smell different herbs, and intuitively decide which to use when flavoring the root vegetables. Have fun and be creative. "

Roast a Radish

If you've never roasted a radish, try a few and notice the difference between a spicy raw radish and a sweet roasted radish.

Roots are Good for Us!

Roots are nutrient-dense, grounding, and sweet. Enjoy experimenting with the many different types of roots, such as carrots, celery root, golden beets, red beets, parsnips, sweet potatoes, turnips, and radishes. Root vegetables are:

- Nutrient-dense with calcium, iron, beta carotene, and vitamins A, C, and E.
- Energetically grounding, as roots grow in the earth.
- Naturally sweet when cooked, thus helping reduce sugar cravings.

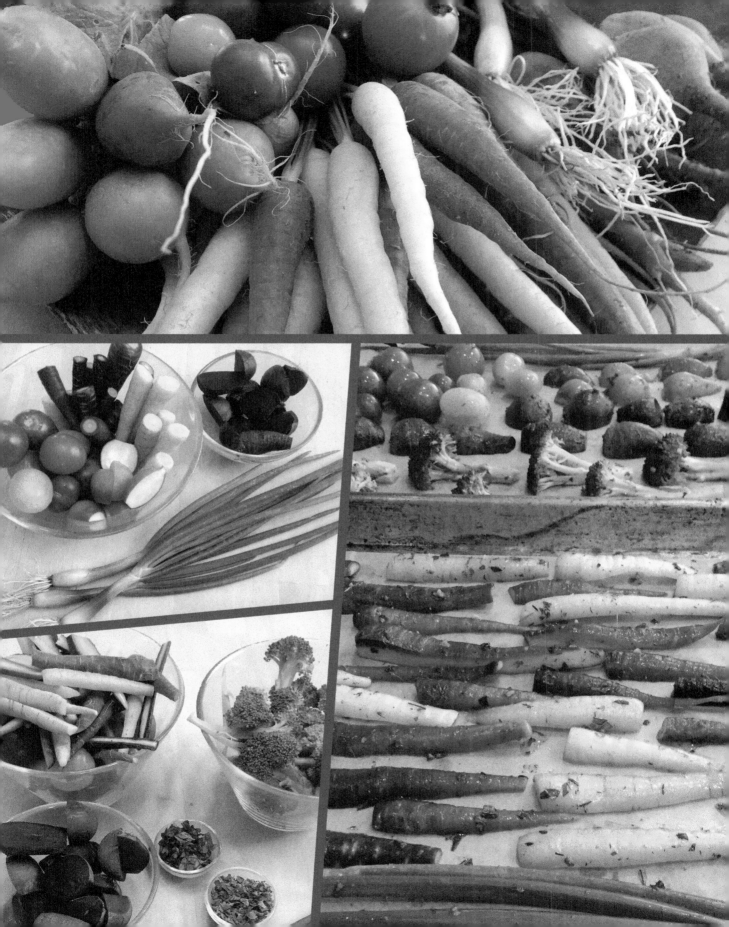

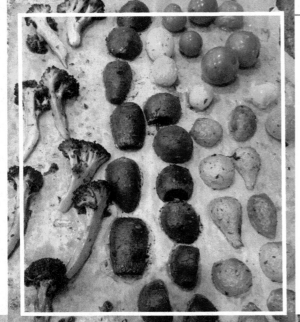

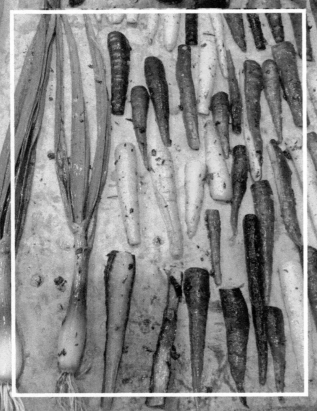

7 Culinary Tips for Great Roasted Roots

1. When roasting roots, the key to creating a crisp, caramelized exterior and a soft interior is to totally coat all sides of the vegetable with olive oil, which helps them brown more easily and not dry out.

2. Season with sea salt to bring out the natural flavors of the roots.

3. Do not dump the roots onto the parchment paper. Instead, mindfully lift the roots out of the bowl and place them onto the tray. Too much oil on the tray will result in steaming rather than roasting.

4. Use compostable unbleached chlorine-free parchment paper. The caramelized bits from the root stay on the food rather than the sheet pan. Plus, parchment paper is ideal for the environment, no greasing is necessary, and it's easy to clean-up.

5. Roast each vegetable separately, as they all cook at different rates.

6. Place the baking sheet in the middle of the oven for even heat distribution around the vegetables.

7. Serve roasted vegetables in a shallow dish so that they do not steam.

5 Ways to Finish Roasted Roots

To make root vegetables interesting, experiment with different ways to finish them.

1. Sprinkle flavored sea salt for a unique taste.
2. Drizzle oil to add sheen,
3. Squeeze fresh citrus: lemon, lime, or orange for zestiness.
4. Add toasted nuts or seeds for a little crunch.
5. Add fresh herbs to create a fresh taste.

Action

Once you've learned the roasted roots cooking technique, experiment by roasting with other vegetables, such as asparagus, broccoli, Brussels sprouts, and cauliflower. Enjoy the deep, rich, roasted flavors of these veggies.

Slow-Roasted Golden Beets in a Bag

Create gourmet, vegetarian, restaurant-quality beets in your kitchen with a few simple ingredients – beets, fresh lemon, oil, herbs, and salt – and impress your family and friends with your creation. Enjoy this slow cooking process that brings out the sweet, earthy flavor of the beets and concentrates the beet flavor with the citrus of the lemon.

SIMPLE INGREDIENTS

- 4-5 medium beets, whole and unpeeled
- ¼ cup vegetable stock
- 1 lemon, juiced and sliced rind
- 2 sprigs fresh thyme
- Dressing: Your choice, with a fat, acid, and salt.

SIMPLE STEPS

1. Gather your mise en place.
2. Preheat oven to 275 degrees F.
3. Scrub the beets well.
4. In a medium bowl, toss beets with vegetable stock, lemon juice, and thyme sprigs.
5. Wrap the beets, vegetable stock, and lemon juice in a tent with natural parchment paper, leaving room for the beets to steam. Tighten edges of the parchment paper tent.
6. Place the tent on a sheet pan and cook for 45-60 minutes.
7. Test the beets for doneness. They are ready when fork-tender.
8. If peeling beets, do not peel underwater, as they will lose some of the flavor gained from cooking.
9. To finish the dish, cut the beets and toss with a simple dressing.
10. Serve as a side dish, in a salad, or as an appetizer with Raw Cashew Cream.

Be Creative with Beets in a Bag

Have fun experimenting with different fresh herbs, such as basil, lemon balm, lemon thyme, oregano, or thyme.

Raw Cashew Cream

Dairy-free nut cream is a great substitute for cheese and is a beautiful base for the Slow-Roasted Golden Beets. Make a batch of the base cream and add your favorite herbs and aromatics for a tasty dip, or spread for raw veggies or crackers.

SIMPLE INGREDIENTS

- 2 cups raw cashews, soaked
- 2 tbsp lemon juice
- Water, just enough to blend the cashews
- 2 tbsp nutritional yeast
- 1 tsp onion granules
- Extras: Fresh chopped herbs (basil, parsley, dill), minced aromatics (green onions, chives, shallot)

SIMPLE STEPS

1. Place cashews in a bowl, cover with water, and soak for 3-4 hours or overnight.
2. To make the nut spread, blend cashews with lemon juice and just enough water to blend into a smooth consistency.
3. Add nutritional yeast and onion granules, and stir to combine.
4. Mix in your favorite extras with fresh herbs or aromatics.
5. Serve as a base for Slow Roasted Golden Beets, with raw crackers, as a veggie dip, or as a spread for a wrap.

> **"** I get excited about food. I love the natural beauty of food at farmers' markets, and how outstanding fresh, recently harvested, locally grown food is when we take the time to mindfully prepare and cook it. This beet dish has totally exceeded my expectations for a side dish, with the rich earthiness of the beets combined with the sharp zest of the lemon. **"**

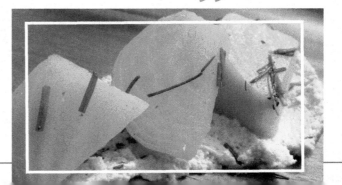

SWEET POTATO AND CHICKPEA BURGERS WITH ROASTED RED PEPPERS

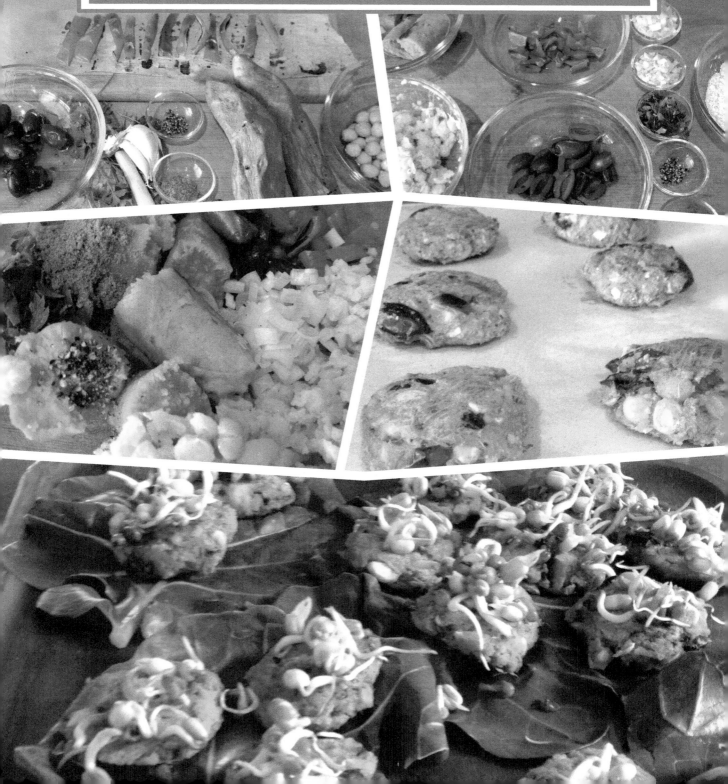

These tasty burger-like patties are a fun, mindful way to cook mini-burgers for lunch, snacks, or appetizers. This recipe is doubled, so you can make a big batch and freeze some of the burgers for snacks. The recipe makes 12 burgers or 24 mini-burgers.

SIMPLE INGREDIENTS

- 2 large sweet potatoes, baked whole, 2 cups cooked
- 1 cup chickpeas, cooked and coarsely mashed
- ½ cup Kalamata olives, sliced
- ½ cup roasted red peppers
- ½ cup rolled oats, ground into meal

- 6 tbsp red onion, minced
- 2 tbsp onion powder
- 4 cloves garlic, minced
- 6 tbsp fresh parsley, finely chopped
- 1 tsp cumin seeds, hand-ground into powder
- ½ tsp freshly ground black pepper

SIMPLE STEPS

1. Gather your mise en place.
2. Bake sweet potato. Once baked, peel off the skin.
3. To prepare the burger mixture, toss together all ingredients except the oats, pressing the potato until the mixture begins to bind. If the mixture is too moist, mix in the oats.
4. Form the mixture into burger-size patties or bite-size appetizers and place on a parchment paper-lined baking sheet.
5. Bake for 15 minutes, flip, and bake for another 5-8 minutes until both sides are golden.
6. Serve on a raw cracker, in a wrap with roasted veggies, or on a collard green leaf with sprouted mung beans. Steam the collard greens for a few minutes in a bamboo steamer.
7. Store cooked leftover sweet potato chickpea burgers, separated by parchment paper, in the freezer. Reheat in an oven at 325 degrees until defrosted and warm.

" These sweet potato burgers are one of those recipes where it is important to be organized in your kitchen and to set up your mise en place to help make your cooking process easy. There are a lot of ingredients, and you must cook the sweet potatoes and chickpeas before making the burgers, so get organized and have fun making this veggie burger. "

7 Steps to Bake Sweet Potatoes

1. Preheat oven to 400 degrees F.
2. Puncture sweet potatoes with a fork.
3. Place onto parchment-lined baking sheet.
4. Bake for 35-50 minutes, depending on the size of the sweet potatoes.
5. Potatoes are ready when a fork slides through the center with ease.
6. Cool for 5-10 minutes.
7. Use sweet potatoes in your recipe, or enjoy eating with your meal or as a snack.

SIMPLE VEGGIE STIR-FRY WITH ROOTS AND IN-SEASON PRODUCE

One of my favorite ways to cook all kinds of vegetables, including roots, is a simple stir-fry (really a simple sauté) with what's seasonally available from local farmers. The beautiful veggies available during the first week of my winter 2016 CSA (Community Supported Agriculture) from Maya's Farm at the Farm at South Mountain, only a mile from my Phoenix home, inspired this intuitive stir-fry.

To create a simple veggie stir-fry, chose a few local in-season veggies, some roots and some greens. This stir-fry was inspired by the baby bok choy and fresh green garlic in my CSA. Added to the stir-fry were other veggies from local farmers, along with sun-dried tomatoes and capers. During the middle of the stir-fry, I decided to de-glaze the pan with fresh lemon and to add local Arizona citrus to the dish.

SIMPLE INGREDIENTS

- Organic extra virgin olive oil
- Green garlic
- Brussels sprouts
- Carrots
- Cauliflower
- Sun-dried tomatoes
- Capers
- Asparagus
- Baby bok choy
- Sea salt
- Fresh lemon

SIMPLE STEPS

1. Gather your mise en place.
2. Pre-heat sauté pan on medium-high.
3. Pour organic extra virgin olive oil into the pan.
4. Add the aromatics (green garlic) and cook a few minutes.
5. Toss in veggies you'd like to brown a little (Brussels sprouts).
6. Add dense vegetables that need to cook a bit longer (carrots, cauliflower).
7. Toss in extras (sun-dried tomatoes, capers).
8. Add vegetables that do not need to cook very long (asparagus, bok choy).
9. Enjoy!

What's the Difference: Sauté vs. Stir-fry

Sautéing and stir-frying are similar dry-heat cooking methods to cook bite-size pieces of food quickly over high heat. Use a pan to sauté and a wok to stir-fry. With stir-frying, the heat is higher and the action is faster with the food continuously tossed and stirred.

" Have fun preparing quick, delicious veggie stir-fries with a few simple steps. The key is to be organized. Pre-chop all your ingredients and set up your mise en place (all ingredients in place) for your cooking before you start stir-frying. "

Action : Experiment with Roots

In this section, we've explored very different ways of cooking roots: steaming in a bamboo steamer, roasting in a hot oven, steaming in parchment paper, creating a root-based veggie burger, and creating a stir-fry with local farmers' vegetables. I invite you to experiment with one culinary method of cooking roots. Use your intuition when you shop and creatively prepare your roots dish.

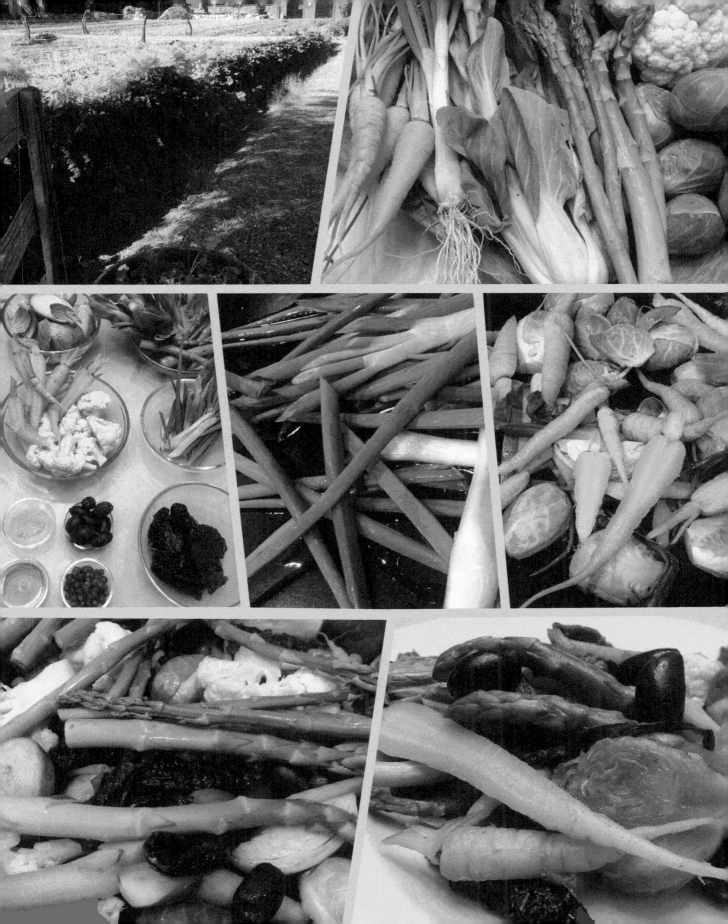

Create Your Own Stir-fry with Local In-Season Organic Roots & Veggies

Asparagus, Snap Peas & Dill

Rainbow Carrots, Golden Beets & Brussels Sprouts

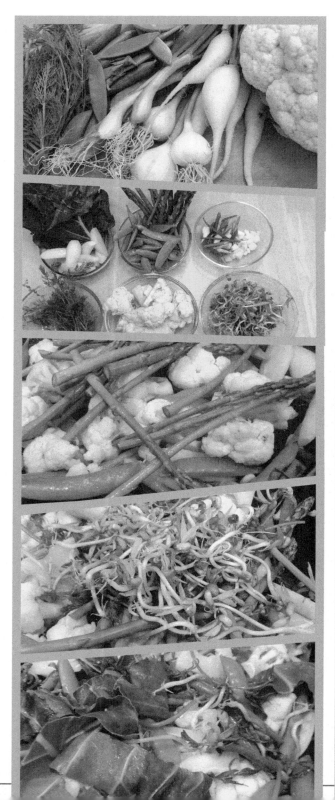

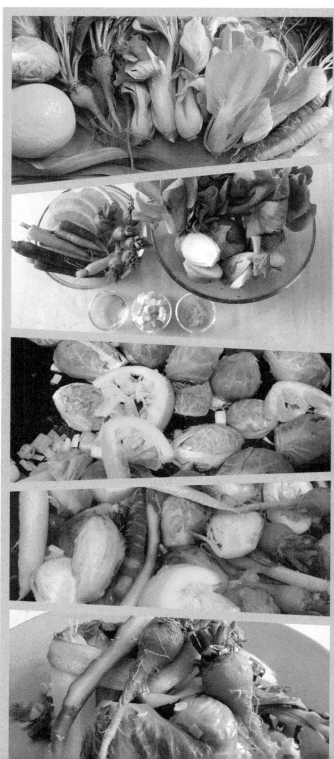

Beets, Broccoli & Brussels Sprouts

Rainbow Carrots & Golden Beets

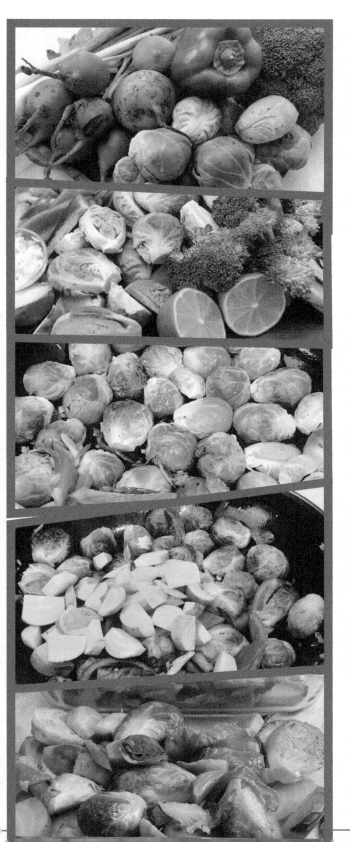
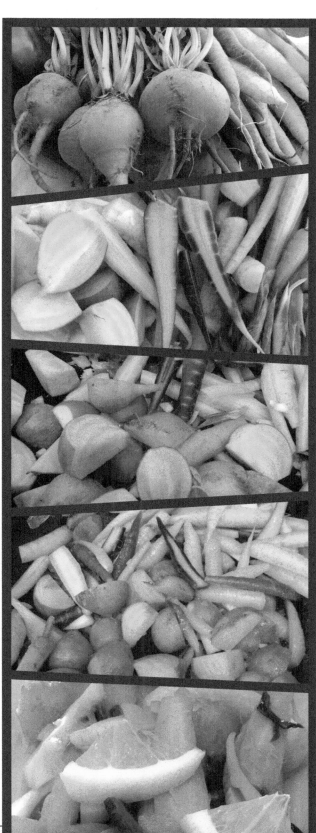

Add Protein-Rich Legumes to Meals

Culinary

- Popular legumes
- How to enjoy beans
- Get creative with your own hummus
- 2 ways to cook beans
- How to tenderize beans
- 7 culinary tips to make beans part of your weekly menu
- How to shop for high-quality canned tomatoes
- How to mindfully enjoy spices & herbs
- 7 simple steps to sprout mung beans

Recipes

- EXPERIENCE NUTRITION™ Super Simple Organic Hummus
- Chickpeas with Sun-dried Tomatoes and Kale
- EXPERIENCE NUTRITION™ Lentil Soup with Sweet Roots & Greens
- Lentil San Marzano Tomato Soup
- Walnut Kidney Bean Chili

Nutrition

- Why protein is essential
- Top plant sources of protein
- Get clear on complete and incomplete proteins
- Tips for vegetarians and vegan to eat complete protein
- Leaders in the plant-based way of eating

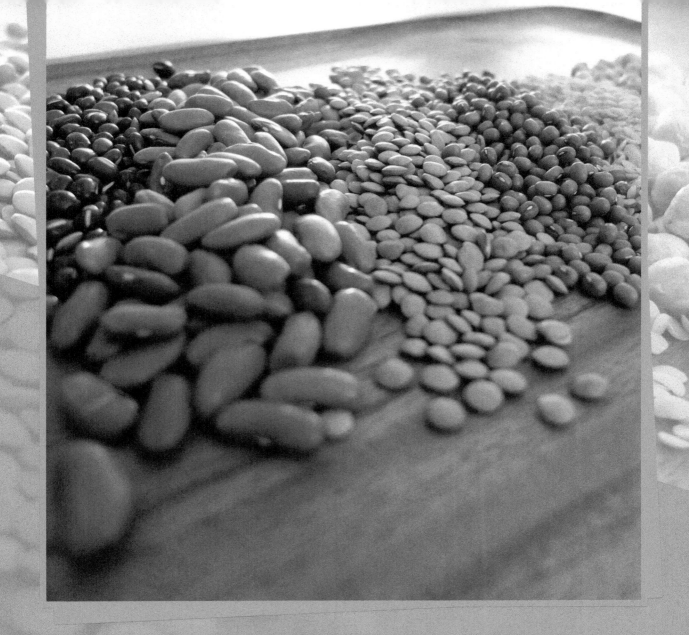

ADD PROTEIN-RICH LEGUMES TO MEALS

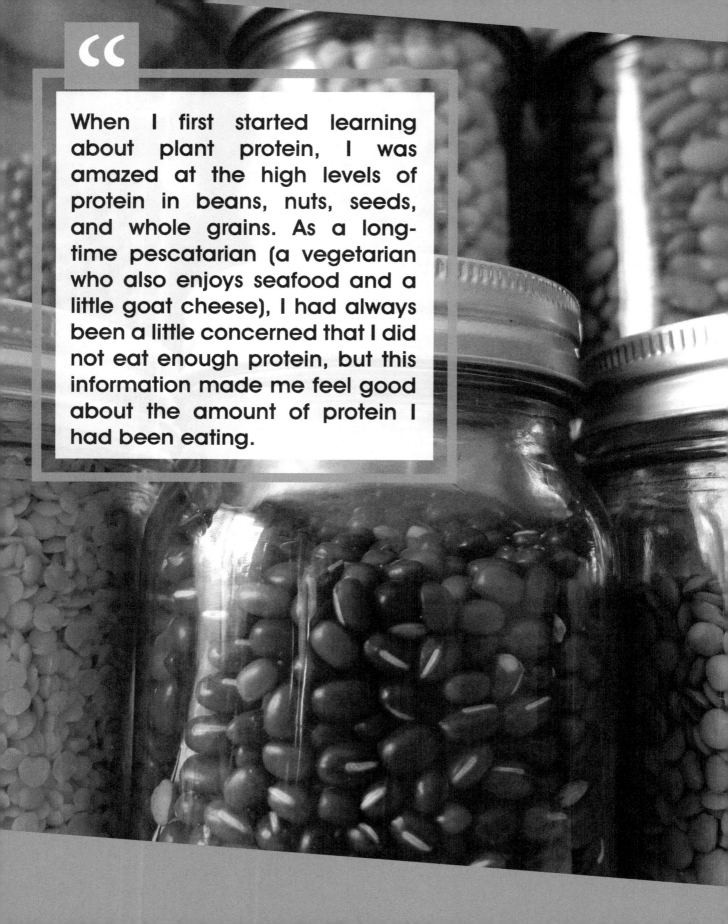

"

When I first started learning about plant protein, I was amazed at the high levels of protein in beans, nuts, seeds, and whole grains. As a long-time pescatarian (a vegetarian who also enjoys seafood and a little goat cheese), I had always been a little concerned that I did not eat enough protein, but this information made me feel good about the amount of protein I had been eating.

ADD PROTEIN-RICH LEGUMES TO MEALS

We must eat protein every day

Protein, along with fats and carbohydrates, is a macronutrient that we must consume every day, ideally at every meal. Protein is a building block for our body; it's the foundation of bones, muscles, cartilage, skin, and blood. Our bodies use protein to build and repair tissues and to make enzymes, hormones, and other body chemicals.

Getting clear on plants that are rich in protein and learning how to prepare simple, delicious recipes with key plant proteins – like beans and lentils – in hummus, soup, and chili gives us a way to easily add protein to our lives.

In this section you will learn how to:

- Why protein is essential
- Top plant sources of protein
- Leaders in the plant-based way of eating

You'll learn how to:

- Cook chickpeas (garbanzo beans) and tenderize them.
- Make hummus, just like the hummus we served at the VIP Tailgate Party at Super Bowl XLIV in Miami.
- Sauté chickpeas with sun-dried tomatoes and kale for a simple plant-based meal.
- Make lentil and sweet potato soup as the foundation for all kinds of bean soup.
- Cook lentil tomato soup with San Marzano tomatoes.
- Create walnut kidney bean chili that even meat eaters will enjoy.
- Sprout mung beans.

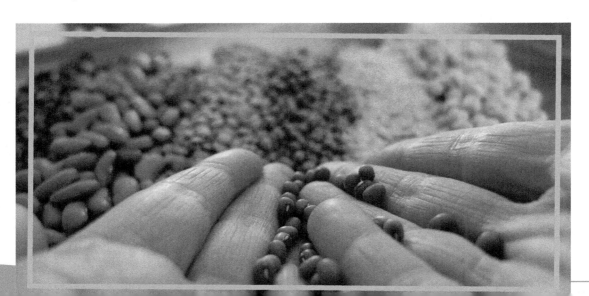

GET TO KNOW PROTEIN

I stopped eating meat 30 years ago because my body could not digest it. I was a runner and intuitively felt (in my body) that the meat made me sluggish. Then 20 years ago when my mom was diagnosed with breast cancer, I learned about the antibiotics in poultry and stopped eating turkey and chicken, which I loved at the time.

For years, my family was worried that I was not eating enough protein, and I didn't know how to cook meals without meat or poultry at the center of the plate. While I was studying at the Institute for Integrative Medicine in New York in 2006-2007, I learned so much about "good" plant proteins, such as beans, lentils, nuts, seeds, grains, and even some vegetables.

When teaching former NFL players and their families to cook, it was important to cook plant proteins, so I learned simple, basic ways to cook beans and lentils. I've now been sharing the simple legumes cooking techniques for nearly 10 years.

We Get Protein from Plants and Animals

Top protein-rich plants include:
- Legumes (beans, lentils, peas)
- Nuts and seeds
- Whole grains
- Sea vegetables

Top animal sources of protein are:
- Meat
- Fish
- Poultry
- Cheese

Protein in Plants and Animals

A few years ago, when guiding former NFL players and their families about nutrition and cooking, I created this Simple Protein Chart from the USDA database to examine the level of protein in different types of food and to compare plant and animal protein sources. When we clearly examine protein sources, we see that we can indeed get enough protein in our diets from plant-based foods rather than from the typical SAD – Standard American Diet – of red meat, pork, poultry, and dairy.

It's important to note how the levels of protein in many plant foods are comparable to the protein levels in meat, poultry, cheese, and fish. For instance, in a 3.5-ounce serving, pork and tuna have 30 grams, and chicken and Swiss cheese both contain 27 grams of protein. These levels of protein in animal food are comparable to pumpkin seeds with 30 grams, lentils with 26 grams, and hemp seeds with 23 grams.

> " When I look at this protein list, I am happy to see that many protein-rich plants are foods I eat every week. Personally, I eat lots of nuts (almonds and cashews), seeds (pumpkin, sunflower, and hemp), beans (garbanzo and lentils), snacks (raw cacao and goji berries), and quinoa. "

 Reasons Why Protein is Essential
- It is a macro-nutrient, which our bodies require every day.
- It builds and repairs tissues.
- It makes enzymes, hormones, and other body chemicals.

 Tips to Eat the Right Amount of Protein
- About 25 percent of our daily diet should come from protein.
- Eat protein at every meal.
- The average serving size of protein fits in the palm of your hand.

 Reasons Why Protein is Extra Important for Athletes
- It stimulates metabolism.
- It improves muscle mass and recovery.
- It reduces body fat.

Simple Protein Chart

Protein Grams per 100 Grams (3.53-ounce) servings

30.2 Pumpkin seeds	20.3 Pistachio nuts
30.0 Pork	19.4 Beef, grass-fed, ground
30.0 Tuna	
29.1 Beef tenderloin steak, lean only	19.3 Garbanzo beans, raw
	19.3 Sunflower seeds
29.3 Turkey	18.3 Flax seeds
28.4 Nori (sea vegetable)	18.2 Cashews
27.3 Salmon, sockeye	18.1 Beef tenderloin
27.1 Chicken	16.6 Soybeans
26.9 Swiss cheese	16.6 Inca berries*
26.7 Halibut	16.5 Chia seeds
26.7 Beef chuck eye roast	15.4 Cacao*
25.8 Lentils, raw	15.2 Walnuts
23.6 Kidney beans, raw	14.3 Goji berries
22.5 Hemp seeds	14.1 Quinoa, uncooked
21.6 Black beans, raw	12.4 Cottage cheese, 1% fat
21.5 Dulse (sea vegetable)	
21.4 Pinto beans, raw	3.4 Milk, non-fat
21.2 Almonds	3.3 Soymilk

Source: USDA National Nutrient Database
* Not in USDA Database

Get Clear on Complete and Incomplete Proteins

While there are high levels of protein in some plants, it's important to also explore how plant protein compares to animal protein in terms of amino acids, the building blocks of all proteins. A complete protein consists of all nine essential amino acids. Our bodies cannot make essential amino acids on their own, so we must eat food with amino acids every day for optimum health.

Animal Protein is a complete protein with all essential amino acids. Animal sources of protein, such as meat, chicken, milk, fish, eggs, and dairy, tend to be complete.

Most Plant Proteins are incomplete. Most vegetarian sources of protein lack one or more essential amino acids; that is, amino acids that the body can't make from scratch or create by modifying another amino acid. Most fruits, vegetables, grains, and nuts are incomplete proteins.

Tips for Vegetarians or Vegans to Eat Complete Protein

It is possible for vegetarians or vegans – who don't eat meat, poultry, eggs, dairy, or fish – to eat complete proteins.

- **Eat foods that are complete proteins.** Soy, amaranth, hemp seeds, chia seeds, quinoa, and buckwheat.

- **Eat a variety of protein-rich foods.** Nuts, legumes, whole grains, fruit, and vegetables, which, when combined, create a complete protein.

- **Enjoy a meal with a whole grain and beans or lentils.** Staple meals in many parts of the world naturally combine whole grains and legumes. Think rice and beans or pita and hummus.

A Blue Zone: The Nicoya Peninsula, Costa Rica

A few years ago, I spent a few months coaching clients about nutrition at the spa at The Harmony Hotel in Nosara, Costa Rica. I was fortunate to spend time living in one of the Blue Zones, where people live the longest, and I experienced the typical rice and beans with many meals.

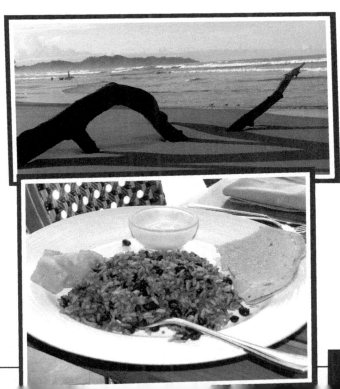

GET TO KNOW LEGUMES: BEANS, LENTILS, AND PEAS

Legumes, plants that have pods containing small seeds, include beans, lentils, peas, and a few nuts. Legumes are eaten around the world, and there are many different types to enjoy as a side dish or the core of a meal.

Popular Legumes

- **Beans:** Adzuki, black, cannellini, fava, garbanzo, kidney, lima, navy, pinto, soy
- **Lentils:** Black, brown, green, orange, red, yellow
- **Peas:** Black-eyed, green, snow, snap, split

Because legumes are rich in protein, they are the perfect option for vegetarians, vegans, and people who want to limit their consumption of meat or poultry. Half a cup of beans provides about 6-7 grams of protein, which is about the same as 1 ounce of meat, poultry, or fish.

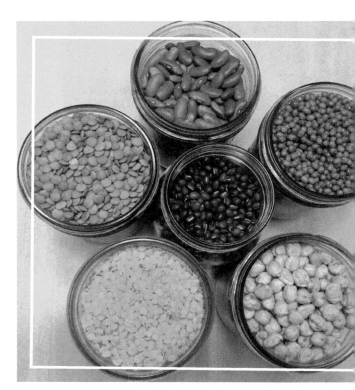

In addition to being protein-rich, beans are a good source of fiber. High-fiber diets are associated with lower risks of heart disease, diabetes, obesity, and cancer. Regarding heart health, beans are rich in soluble fiber, which can lower cholesterol and triglyceride levels. High-fiber foods like beans are also low-glycemic, meaning that they raise blood sugar levels very slowly and, as a result, help regulate blood sugar and lower the risk of diabetes.

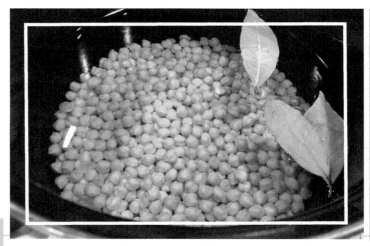

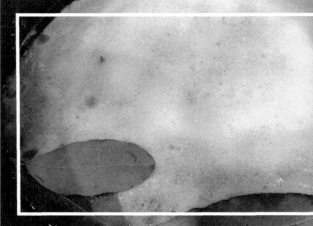

One of the important first steps in eating plant protein is to learn how to cook beans, which are full of both protein and fiber. With a little preparation, beans are very simple to cook and much more cost efficient than canned beans. They also add texture and flavor to dishes.

These two cooking methods work well for large beans, such as adzuki, black, cannellini (white kidney), garbanzo, great northern, kidney, mung, navy, pinto, and soybeans. We do not need to pre-cook small legumes such as lentils and split peas, which can be used directly in a dish.

To start cooking dried beans, purchase firm, clean beans. The exterior should be shiny, as dull beans may be old. Store beans in a cool, dark place, such as a dark pantry.

Way 1: Soak Beans: When you remember to pre-soak the beans

Soaking re-hydrates beans, reduces cooking time, and improves digestibility.

1. Soak beans at least 8 hours with at least twice as much cold water as the beans. Soak on your counter or, if your kitchen is warm, in the refrigerator.
2. After the beans have re-hydrated, drain and rinse with cold water.
3. Put beans into a pot with about twice as much new cold water.
4. Add kombu (a sea vegetable) or bay leaves to tenderize the beans.
5. Cover pot and bring to a boil.
6. Skim off the foam (sugar releasing from the beans) that rises to the top of the pot to help reduce flatulence.
7. Lower heat and simmer for 30 minutes to 2 hours with the lid ajar. The length of time for cooking depends on the size of the beans, the age of the beans, and how long they have soaked.
8. If adding salt to the beans, add it halfway through the cooking process.
9. During cooking, test the beans for doneness. They should be creamy – not mushy or crunchy – on the inside.
10. Pour off cooking water, saving any that you may need in your recipe, such as hummus, or for stock.

Way 2: When you forget to pre-soak the beans

When we forget to pre-soak beans we can cook them, but the cooking time is longer than it is with pre-soaked beans.

1. Put beans into a pot with at least twice as much cold water as the beans, along with kombu or bay leaves.
2. Boil for 2-3 minutes.
3. Turn off heat, cover, and let sit for 1-4 hours.
4. Drain and rinse beans.
5. Put beans back into pot with about twice as much cold water.
6. Cover pot and bring to a boil.
7. Skim off foam that rises to the top.
8. Lower heat and simmer for 2-3 hours with the lid ajar.
9. Pour off cooking water, saving any that you may need in your recipe, such as hummus, or for stock.

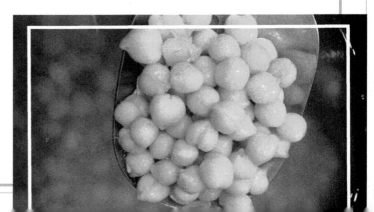

MAKE YOUR OWN HUMMUS: EXPERIENCE NUTRITION™ SUPER SIMPLE ORGANIC HUMMUS

I'm excited to share with you the same recipe we made for the Super Bowl XLIV VIP Tailgate Party for the Super Bowl in Miami. Now you can make it, too.

SIMPLE INGREDIENTS

- 2 cups cooked chickpeas (garbanzo beans)
- $\frac{1}{3}$ cup chickpea water
- 3 tbsp tahini (sesame seed paste or sesame seeds)
- 3 cloves garlic
- 2 tbsp fresh lemon juice
- $\frac{1}{4}$ tsp black pepper
- $\frac{1}{8}$ tsp cumin seeds, ground
- $\frac{1}{8}$ tsp coriander seeds, ground (seeds from cilantro)

SIMPLE STEPS

1. Place all ingredients into high-speed blender (such as Vitamix) or food processor.
2. Blend until smooth.
3. After the hummus has been blended, taste and add more of any of the ingredients to suit your taste.

How to Enjoy Beans

- **Slowly introduce beans to your diet.** As with all fiber-rich foods, introduce legumes slowly into your diet to allow time for your digestive system to adapt.
- **Start with smaller legumes.** If you are new to legumes, start with lentils and split peas, which are easier to digest and do not need to be soaked.
- **Experiment in cooking.** Beans are so versatile and can be eaten so many different ways. Eat beans simply with a whole grain and green veggie, add to a salad, use them in soup or chili, or eat hummus as a snack.

Get Creative with Hummus

Make your own version of hummus. Once you've learned how to make the basic hummus, have fun experimenting and intuitively creating your own versions of it.

- **Interesting extras.** Add any of the following and blend again or gently fold into the hummus: Cilantro, basil, dill, roasted peppers, sun-dried tomatoes, olives, or sautéed onions and garlic.

- **Different beans.** Be creative and make hummus with various kinds of beans, such as black beans, navy beans, or a combination of your favorite beans.

- **Tahini or sesame seeds.** Experiment with pre-made tahini, or hand-grind your own sesame seeds in a mortar and pestle.

- **World flavors.** Experiment with different herbs and spices. Make Mediterranean hummus with basil, oregano, marjoram, roasted red peppers, olives, and capers. Try Mexican hummus with chili powder, coriander, garlic, fresh Jalapeno peppers, and cilantro. Create an Indian version with cumin, cardamom, cinnamon, and ginger.

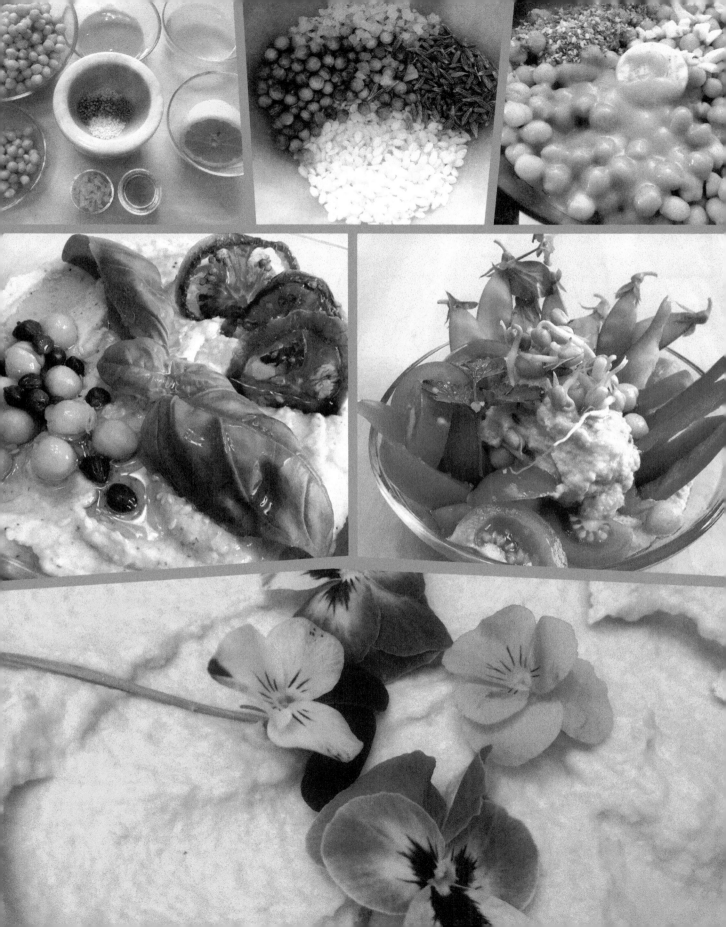

EXPERIENCE NUTRITION™ LENTIL SOUP WITH SWEET ROOTS AND GREENS

This soup cooking process gives you the culinary foundation to cook any type of bean or lentil soup. To make quick, delicious soups, you will use a mix-and-match of legumes, roots, whole grains, and greens.

- **Legumes:** Lentils, black beans, navy beans, pinto beans
- **Roots:** Carrots, parsnips, sweet potatoes, turnips
- **Whole grains:** Brown rice, quinoa
- **Greens:** Kale, collards, spinach

SIMPLE INGREDIENTS

- 1 cup lentils
- 3-4 carrots and/or sweet potatoes, chopped
- 2-3 cloves garlic, minced
- 1 onion or 5-6 green onions, minced
- 3-4 celery stalks, chopped
- 2 tbsp organic extra virgin olive oil
- 5-inch strip of kombu seaweed
- 1 cup brown rice or quinoa
- 4-6 cups water
- ½ tsp cumin seeds, hand-ground
- 1 tsp black pepper
- ½ bunch kale, torn or chopped into bite-size pieces

Former NFL player, John Bronson intuitively created his Lentil Soup with Sweet Potatoes and Turmeric.

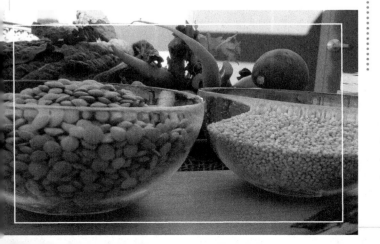

SIMPLE STEPS

1. Gather your mise en place.
2. Pre-heat soup pot over low-medium heat.
3. Add olive oil and onions to the pot.
4. Sweat onions for about 10 minutes, until translucent.
5. Add garlic and cook for about a minute.
6. Add carrots, sweet potatoes, and celery.
7. Increase heat to medium and sauté for about 5 minutes.
8. Add about 4-6 cups of water.
9. Add lentils and whole grain (brown rice or quinoa) to pot.
10. Add ground cumin seeds and black pepper.
11. Increase heat and bring to a boil.
12. Skim off foam that rises to the top.
13. Simmer at low-medium heat for about 30-45 minutes.
14. Sprinkle kale over top of soup and cook 5 more minutes.
15. Enjoy!

> Lentil Soup with Sweet Roots & Greens is absolutely one of my favorites. It's a simple-to-cook comfort food, deliciously sweet, and versatile. Use the recipe as a culinary foundation to create all kinds of bean and whole grain soups.

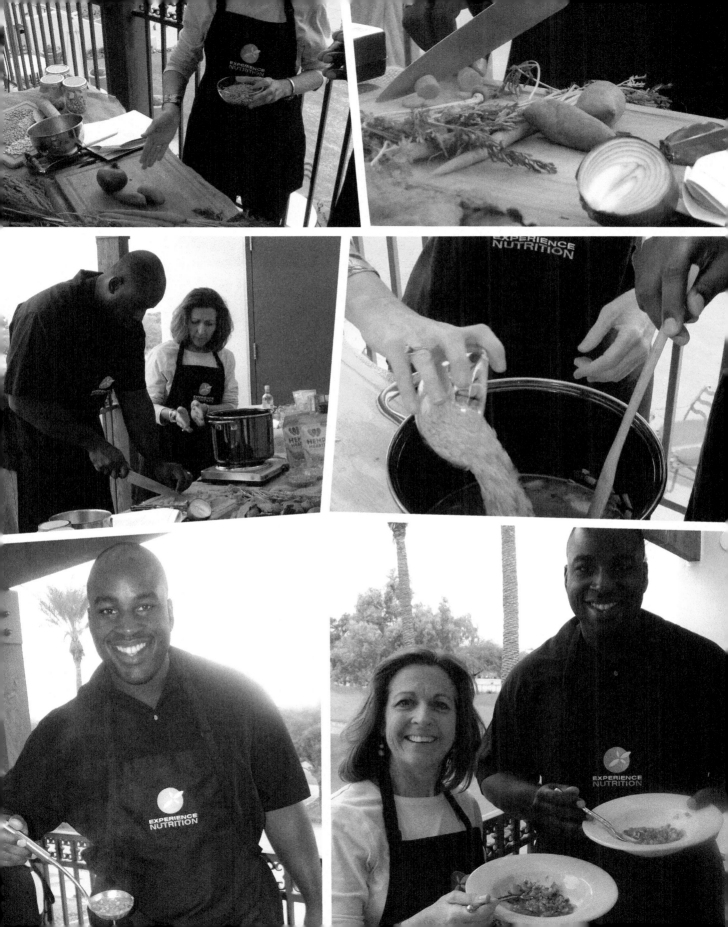

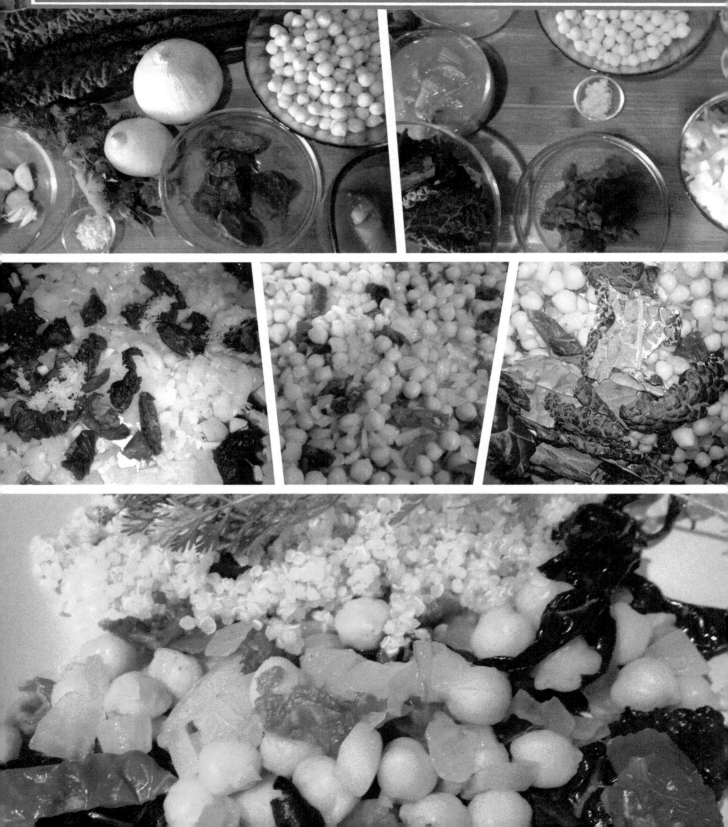

Mindfully craft a beautiful dish with chickpeas (garbanzo beans) for a family gathering or potluck. Enjoy this simple-to-prepare dish that brings basic garbanzo beans to life. While cooking this recipe, enjoy the mindfulness and aromatherapy of sweating onions, garlic, and fresh ginger root. Also, enjoy the experience of transforming simple chickpeas into a beautiful meal.

The culinary process to create this dish serves as a foundation for cooking simple beans with extra flavor. Once you've learned to sauté garbanzo beans into a meal, experiment with your own favorite add-ins. Try fresh tomatoes, broccoli, cauliflower, more garlic, or less or no ginger. Make it Mediterranean with olives, basil, oregano, and marjoram, or create a spicy Mexican dish with chili, coriander, and cumin.

7 Culinary Tips to Make Beans Part of Your Weekly Menu

1. **Buy bulk.** Save money by purchasing organic beans in the bulk section of your store.

2. **Soak beans.** Soaking beans before cooking reduces cooking time and improves digestibility.

3. **Fresh water.** Use fresh water to cook the beans, as the soaking water contains difficult-to-digest starches, which may cause flatulence.

4. **Tenderize.** Add a tenderizer when cooking beans to reduce flatulence. Tenderize with kombu, a Japanese sea vegetable that is rich in calcium, iron, and iodine, or use bay leaves, cumin seeds, fennel, or ginger root.

5. **Aromatics.** To enhance the flavor of beans, add aromatics such as fresh garlic or thyme to the soaking or cooking water.

6. **Make once, use twice.** When you cook beans, make a large batch and use them for a few days in different recipes: hummus, soup, chili, salad, or side dishes. You can also freeze cooked beans for six months and use them later.

7. **Canned beans.** If you buy canned beans, look for beans cooked with kombu and no extra salt.

SIMPLE INGREDIENTS

- 1 yellow onion, diced
- 4 cloves garlic, minced
- 1 tbsp fresh ginger root, minced
- 1 whole lemon, juiced
- ½ cup sun-dried tomatoes
- 2 cups cooked chickpeas
- 1 tbsp organic extra virgin olive oil
- 1 bunch kale, torn into bite-size pieces
- Handful fresh cilantro or basil
- Sea salt
- Black pepper

SIMPLE STEPS

1. Gather mise en place.
   - Dice onion, and mince garlic and ginger.
   - Zest and juice lemon.
   - Measure sun-dried tomatoes; drain if packed in oil.
   - Measure cooked chickpeas.
   - Tear kale into bite-size pieces.

2. Sauté the dish.
   - Pre-heat large, deep sauté pan over low heat.
   - Add the olive oil, onions, and pinch of sea salt.
   - Sweat the onions for about 10 minutes.
   - Once soft and translucent, add garlic and ginger; cook for another minute.
   - Add sun-dried tomatoes and lemon zest and cook for another minute or two.
   - Pour chickpeas into the pan and stir to coat in the sun-dried tomato mixture.
   - Turn up the heat slightly to medium and cook a few minutes, allowing the chickpeas to take on a little color.
   - Once the chickpeas are heated through, add the kale and cook until it wilts.
   - To finish the dish, add lemon juice, sea salt, and pepper to the sauté pan and simmer for a few minutes.
   - Serve immediately with brown rice or quinoa; garnish with fresh basil or cilantro.

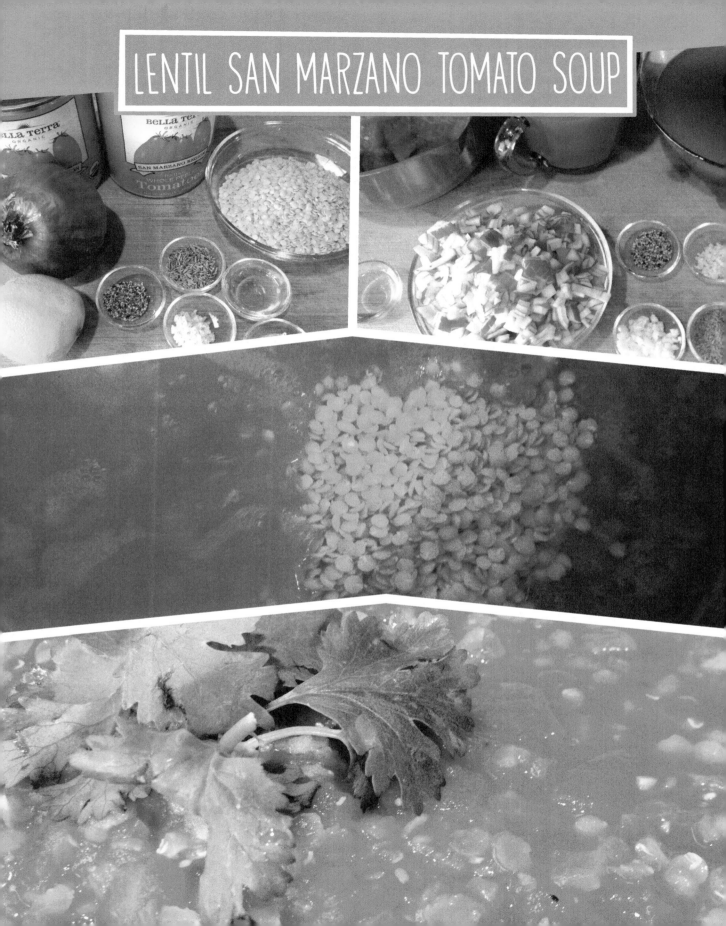

LENTIL SAN MARZANO TOMATO SOUP

Lentil soup with organic San Marzano tomatoes is a beautiful, sweet, rich soup. For this soup, we recommend canned organic San Marzano tomatoes from Italy for high-quality sweet tomatoes year round. With this recipe, enjoy the mindfulness of sweating the onions and garlic, and of prepping the tomatoes and their juice for this simple, incredible soup.

SIMPLE INGREDIENTS

- 1 medium red onion, finely diced
- 3 cloves garlic, minced
- 1 ½ tsp cumin seeds, hand-ground
- 2 28-oz. cans whole organic San Marzano tomatoes
- 1 cup red lentils
- 2 cups vegetable stock
- 1 tbsp organic extra virgin olive oil
- 1 tsp sea salt
- ¼ tsp freshly ground black pepper
- 1 lemon, juiced
- Fresh cilantro, rough chopped

SIMPLE STEPS

1. Prepare your mis en place.
2. Prep tomatoes.
   - To prepare the tomatoes, place a strainer over a bowl, break open each whole tomato, and remove the seeds while allowing the juice to collect in the bowl.
   - Roughly chop the de-seeded tomatoes and place in a bowl.
   - Measure 2 cups of the strained tomato juice and place in another bowl.
3. Cook the soup.
   - Heat a heavy-bottomed large (6- to 8-quart) pot over medium-low heat and add the olive oil.
   - Sweat the onions for about 10 minutes, then add the garlic and cook for about a minute.
   - Add ground cumin seeds and cook until fragrant, about a minute.
   - Add chopped tomatoes, tomato juice, vegetable stock, salt, and pepper and bring to a simmer.
   - Once simmering, add the lentils and simmer until the lentils are cooked, about 20 minutes.
   - If the soup is too thick, add tomato juice or vegetable stock.
   - Garnish with squeezed lemon and freshly chopped cilantro.

" When I looked at my notes from the first time I made this simple lentil soup, my one word was 'Awesome' with a hand-drawn star. Hope you enjoy this soup as much as I do. "

How to Shop for High-Quality Canned Tomatoes

While we generally recommend fresh tomatoes, high-quality sweet Italian tomatoes are perfect for tomato sauces and soups. The top five things to look for in top-quality canned tomatoes are:

1. **Organic San Marzano**. Tomatoes from Italy.
2. **Simple ingredients**. Tomatoes, tomato puree, and/or tomato juice.
3. **No salt or citric acid**. May indicate that the tomatoes were harvested before they were fully ripe.
4. **D.O.P. seal**. Protected Designation of Origin certification guarantees "authentic from Italy" and superior quality.
5. **Bright and firm**. Sweet and rich in flavor.

WALNUT KIDNEY BEAN CHILI

This simple vegan chili with a mix of kidney beans and walnuts is a perfect alternative for meat-eaters. The texture of the walnuts, smoothness of the beans, and freshness of the cilantro together create a delicious vegan chili.

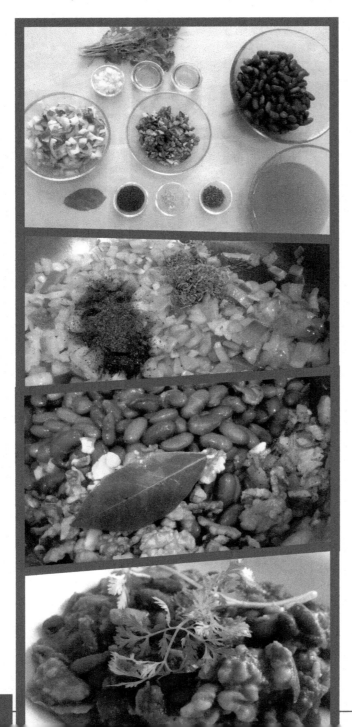

SIMPLE INGREDIENTS

- 1 tbsp extra virgin olive oil
- 1 large onion, diced
- ¼ tsp sea salt
- 3 cloves garlic, minced
- 2 tbsp chili powder
- 1 tsp cumin seeds, hand-ground
- 1 bay leaf
- 2 cups kidney beans, cooked (1 cup dry beans)
- ½ cup raw walnuts, roughly chopped
- 2 cups vegetable stock
- ½ cup cilantro, minced

SIMPLE STEPS

1. Pre-heat 2- to 3-quart soup pot on medium-low heat.
2. Add olive oil, onions and salt; sweat onions for about 10 minutes, until translucent.
3. Add garlic and cook for another minute.
4. Add chili powder and cumin; stir.
5. Add bay leaf, beans, walnuts, and vegetable stock to the onions.
6. Cover and bring to a boil.
7. Reduce heat to low and simmer for about an hour until thick and beans are tender. Add additional stock as needed to moisten and prevent burning.
8. Mash most of the beans with a potato masher in the pot.
9. Cook for 5 additional minutes.
10. Serve topped with fresh cilantro.

3 Fun Ways to Mindfully Enjoy Spices & Herbs

1. **Use a mortar and pestle to hand-grind spices and dried herbs.** Enjoy the mindfulness of hand-grinding and the natural aromatherapy of essential oils in spices and herbs. Try a mix of dry basil, marjoram, and oregano to create a nice Mediterranean blend for roasted root vegetables.

2. **Dry toast spices.** Use a small sauté pan on low heat to lightly toast seeds, such as coriander, cumin, and fennel. Enjoy the aroma and the extra flavor from toasting. Be mindful to cook for only a few minutes so that the spices and seeds do not burn. Toast cumin and coriander seeds to use with bamboo steamer carrots or hummus.

3. **Grate spices by hand.** Enjoy the mindfulness and natural aromatherapy of grinding spices like cinnamon and nutmeg with a hand-held micro-plane grater. Hand-grated spices add extra flavor to desserts, roasted roots, breakfast whole grains, and smoothies.

Plant-Based Leaders

"*The China Study*," by Dr. T Colin Campbell
Twenty-year research study found: "People who ate the most animal-based foods got the most chronic disease. . . People who ate the most plant-based foods were the healthiest and tended to avoid chronic disease."

Brendan Brazier, "*THRIVE: Vegan Nutrition Guide to Optimal Performance in Sports and Life*"
Former professional Ironman triathlete and one of the world's foremost authorities on plant-based nutrition, Brendan Brazier is one of the few professional athletes on an entirely plant-based diet.

"*Forks Over Knives*" Documentary
Feature film examines the claim that most, if not all, of the degenerative diseases that afflict us can be controlled, or even reversed, by rejecting animal-based and processed foods.

John Robbins, "*The Food Revolution: How Your Diet Can Help Save Your Life and Our World*"
In this 2010 food politics classic, learn why John Robbins, the heir to the Baskin-Robbins empire, left his father's business and became a strong proponent of eating a plant-based diet and why he does not recommend eating dairy. According to John Robbins, "The evidence keeps growing that the path to improved health lies in eating more vegetables, fruits, whole grains, and legumes, and eating far less animal products."

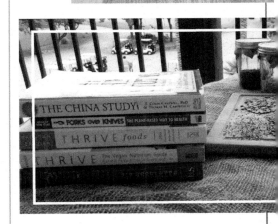

SIMPLY SPROUT BEANS: TRY MUNG BEANS

In the winter of 2014 I started to sprout beans while learning in the Plant-Based Professional Certification with Rouxbe Cooking School. When I visited my parents in Florida, we decided to experiment with sprouting different kinds of organic legumes (mung, adzuki, and green lentils) and a few seeds (sunflower and broccoli). Within a week, we had 12 quart jars full of sprouted beans and seeds. Luckily for my parents' Cocoa Beach neighbors, they also enjoyed sprouts in their meals.

Soaking and Sprouting

The soaking and sprouting process releases dormant enzymes that make beans more easily digestible and, in some cases, even more nutritious.

Mung beans are the most widely eaten sprout on our planet and have been cooked in Chinese dishes for centuries. Mung beans, a great plant protein, are fun and easy to sprout, and can be eaten raw or cooked. Add raw mung beans to the top of a salad, avocado salsa or hummus for a nice crunch. Cook sprouted mung beans for added protein in veggie stir-fries or soup.

Action: Experiment with Plant Protein

In this section, we've explored several ways to enjoy legumes: hummus, lentil soup, chickpeas with sun-dried tomatoes, vegan chili, and sprouting. I invite you to experiment with a few of the culinary methods to prepare legumes. Use your intuition when you shop and creatively prepare your protein-rich meals. Visit us on our Facebook page (www.facebook.com/NewViewHealthyEating) and share your creations.

7 Simple Steps to Sprout Mung Beans

1. Soak ¼ cup dry mung beans in a few cups of water for 8 to 12 hours out of direct sunlight.

2. Rinse beans and place them in a wide-mouth quart Mason jar with a wire lid.

3. Rinse beans with cold water 2 to 4 times a day.

4. After each rinsing, rest the jar on a slant so that any extra water can drain out of the jar. Use a mesh on the lid to allow water to drain.

5. Harvest beans in 2 to 5 days.

6. After sprouts have completely dried, store in the refrigerator.

7. Enjoy raw in a salad or wrap or cooked in a stir-fry.

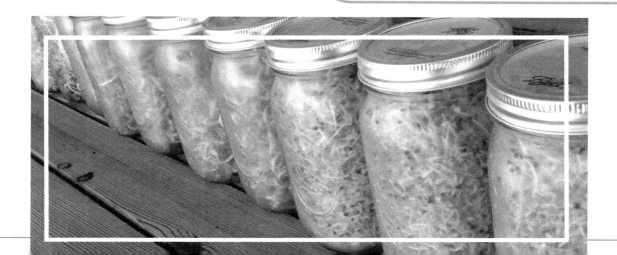

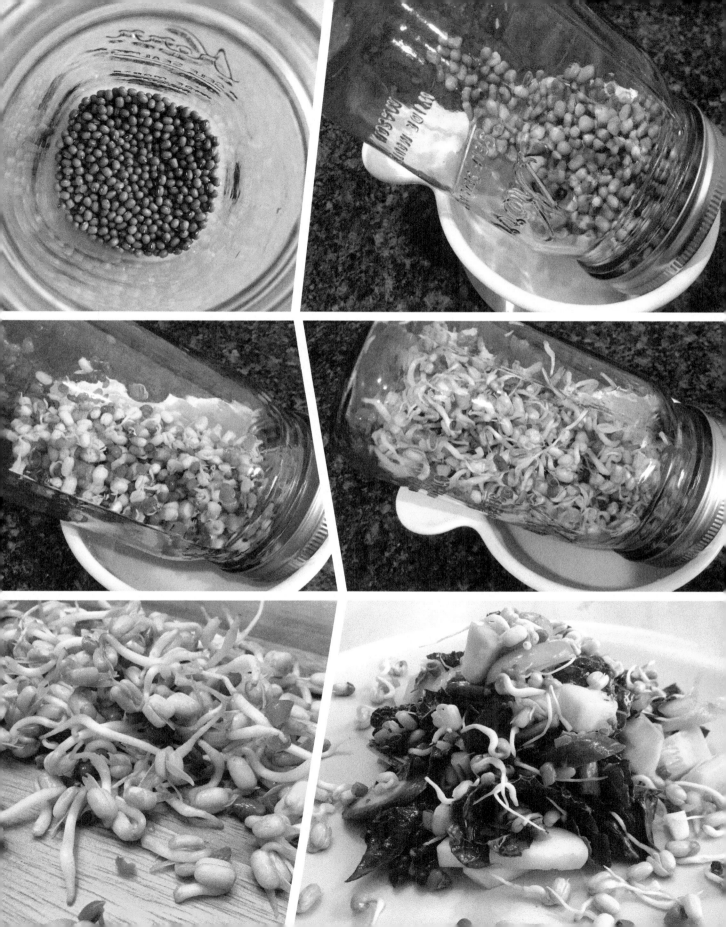

Cook Whole Grains with Simple Culinary Methods

Culinary
- Perfectly cook whole grains on stovetop, oven, and rice cooker
- Tips to make whole grains even better
- Get clear on soaking and rinsing whole grains
- Cook simple steal cut oats breakfast
- Steps to make a variety of veggie burgers
- Cook brown rice pilaf with local veggies
- Prepare brown rice turmeric pilaf
- Experiment with mirepoix
- Tips to make a great risotto
- Steps to par-cook veggies
- How to puree veggies

Recipes
- Simple Steel Cut Oats in Rice Cooker
- Simple Veggie Burgers
- Quick Brown Rice Turmeric Pilaf
- Risotto method: Cook a beautiful, delicious risotto
- Apple Crisp with Oats & Freshly Ground Spices

Nutrition
- Why we need carbs
- Anatomy of a grain
- What makes a grain a whole grain
- Grains from around the world
- Explore pseudograins
- Get clear on gluten

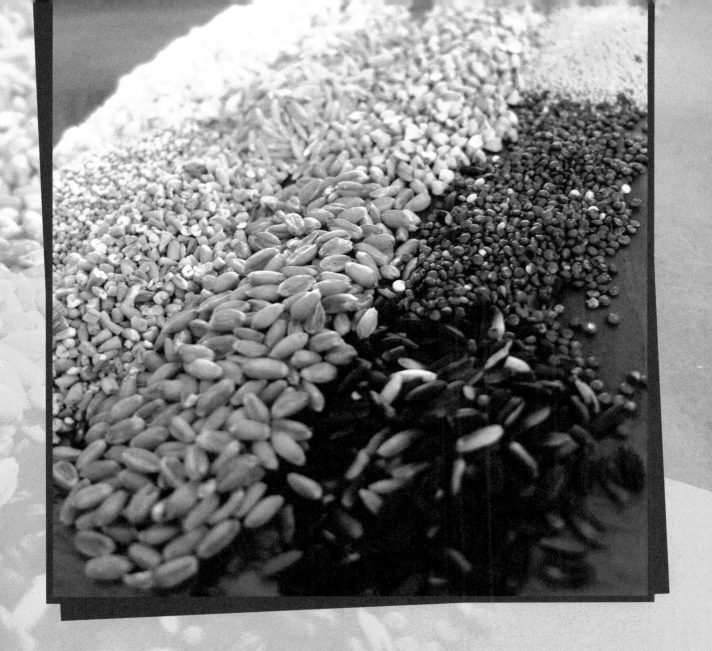

COOK WHOLE GRAINS WITH SIMPLE CULINARY METHODS

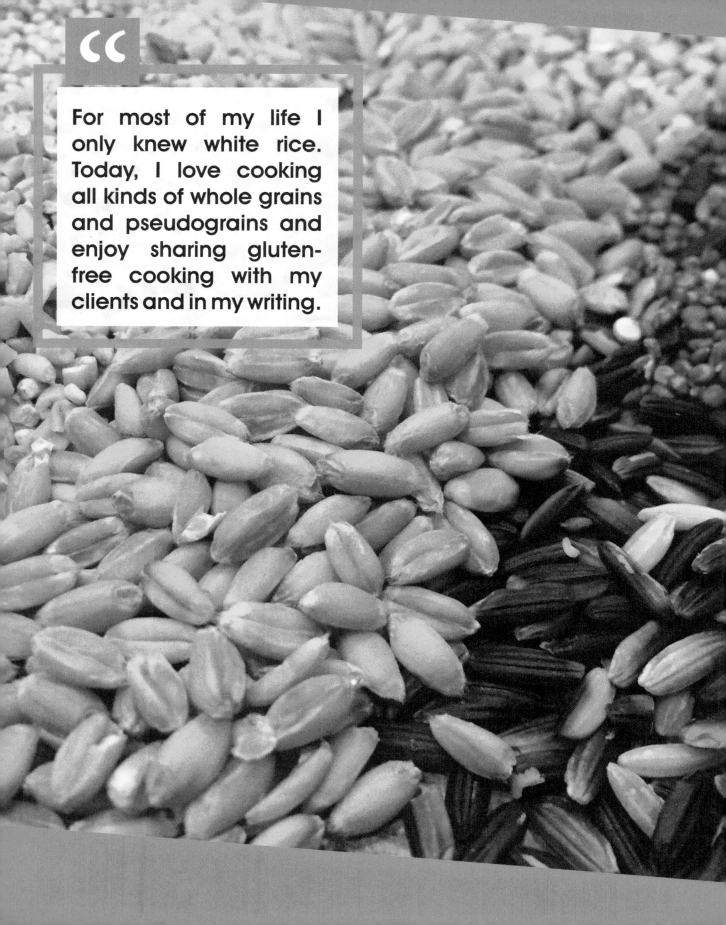

> For most of my life I only knew white rice. Today, I love cooking all kinds of whole grains and pseudograins and enjoy sharing gluten-free cooking with my clients and in my writing.

COOK WHOLE GRAINS WITH SIMPLE CULINARY METHODS

People have been confused about carbs and whole grains for decades

Many believe healthy eating does not include carbs. Many diets are no carb or low carb, but in reality our bodies need about 40-50 percent carbs every day at every meal. The problem is that many people eat low-quality carbs like cookies, cakes, crackers, and bread. Other carbohydrate-rich foods are good for us, including beans, vegetables, and whole grains like brown rice, quinoa, and steel-cut oats.

To get clear on whole grains, we will explore:
- Why we should eat whole grains rather than processed, refined grains
- Grains from around the world
- Gluten sensitivities and celiac disease
- Gluten-free grains

In this section, you'll learn several ways to prepare whole grains so that you can enjoy them at any meal. You'll learn how to:

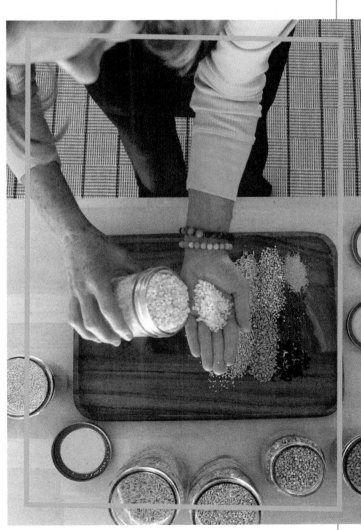

- Perfectly steam whole grains on the stove, in a rice cooker or the oven.
- Cook a quick, simple breakfast with steel-cut oats.
- Make a variety of whole grain burgers.
- Cook brown rice pilaf with local, organic veggies.
- Prepare brown rice turmeric pilaf.
- Cook a beautiful, delicious risotto.
- Bake an incredible, natural, aromatic apple crisp with oats and freshly ground spices.

GET CLEAR ON CARBS AND GRAINS

For most of my life I only knew white rice. Although I had heard about whole grains, I did not incorporate them into my daily eating until I was studying at the Institute for Integrative Nutrition in New York in 2006. At that time, I decided to test for food sensitivities and found that I'm sensitive to gluten, the protein in whole grains, including wheat, barley, and rye.

I stopped eating most food with gluten and now find that when I do eat gluten, I almost immediately react with hives on my skin. I was a little worried about gluten, so I also tested for celiac disease, a serious autoimmune condition in which the body does not absorb nutrients when we eat gluten. Fortunately, I do not have celiac disease.

I'm glad, however, that I've had these experiences, as I can now share gluten-free eating with my clients and in my writing.

Why We Need Carbs

Carbs are:
- The body's primary source of fuel and easily used for energy.
- Needed for the central nervous system, kidneys, brain, and muscles (including the heart) to function properly.
- Stored in the muscles and liver and later used for energy.
- Vital to intestinal health and waste elimination.

Anatomy of a Grain

Our goal is to eat whole grains, which are not processed or refined. It's important to examine the anatomy of a grain to understand the difference between whole grains and grains that are not considered whole grains.

Husk: The hard, non-edible covering of a grain.

Bran: The outer shell of the grain which protects the seed. Bran contains fiber, B vitamins, and minerals.

Germ: Nourishment for the seed. The germ contains B vitamins, minerals, vitamin E, and phytonutrients.

Endosperm: Energy for the seed. The endosperm contains carbohydrates, some protein, and B vitamins.

What's the Difference? Whole, Refined & Enriched Grains

Whole grains: "Good carbs," whole foods which include the germ and bran. Whole grains are not processed. That is, they are not made into other food products like flour, cookies, bread or crackers.

Refined grains: Grains or grain flours that are significantly modified from their natural composition. Refining generally involves mechanical removal of the bran and germ. Further refining includes mixing and bleaching.

Enriched grains: Thiamin, riboflavin, niacin, and iron are often added back to grains to nutritionally enrich them. Because the added nutrients represent a fraction of the nutrients removed, refined grains are considered nutritionally inferior to whole grains.

Why We Need Whole Grains

Consume whole grains

Do not eat grains processed or refined into bread, crackers, or cereal. Whole grains have higher levels of nutrients than refined grains and are protein-rich. Whole grains balance sugar highs and lows. Due to the fiber in whole grains, they digest slowly and produce more stable blood sugar levels than refined, processed grains.

According to the Whole Grains Council (www.WholeGrainsCouncil.org), the benefits of whole grains most documented by studies include:

- Reduce stroke risk by 30-36 percent
- Reduce type 2 diabetes risk by 21-30 percent
- Reduce heart disease risk by 25-28 percent
- Better weight maintenance
- Reduce asthma risk
- Healthier carotid arteries
- Reduce inflammatory disease risk
- Reduce colorectal cancer ris[k]
- Healthier blood pressure leve[ls]
- Less gum disease and tooth loss

Grains from Around the World

Whole grains have been an important part of the diets of many civilizations over time. Today, combinations of grains and legumes – such as lentils and brown rice, black beans and rice, or hummus with pita bread – form the foundation of much of the world's diet. When combined, whole grains and legumes each supply amino acids that the other lack; as a result, when eaten together they offer nutritionally complete protein.

Before you start learning the various culinary methods to cook whole grains, let's explore the different whole grains and pseudograins (grain-like seeds that are protein-rich, gluten-free and typically cooked in a manner similar to whole grains.)

Whole Grains

   Africa: Sorghum (milo)

   Europe: Millet, rice, rye, spelt, wheat

   Middle East: Bulgur, couscous

   Asia & India: Rice

   Ireland & Scotland: Oats

Gluten-Free Pseudograins

   Peru: Quinoa

   Canada: Wild rice

   Mexico: Amaranth

   Russia: Kasha (buckwheat)

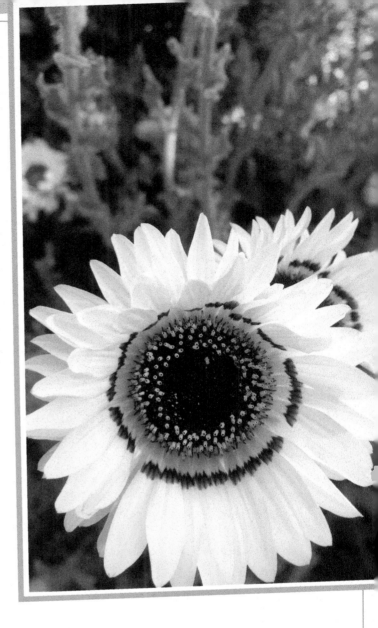

" Pause and enjoy nature. **"**

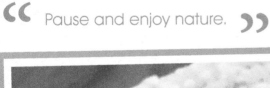

3 FAVORITE WHOLE GRAINS

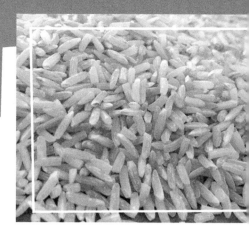

1 Brown Rice: Food Staple Around the World

Brown rice originated in Asia approximately 10,000 years ago and today is one of the most consumed foods in the world. Americans eat about 26 pounds of rice a year; Asians eat as much as 300 pounds, and in France about 10 pounds are consumed.

Only the outer hard covering, the husk, is removed from brown rice, leaving the bran and germ intact. As a result, brown rice has more nutrients and fiber than white rice, which is milled. In white rice, the husk, bran, and germ are all removed, leaving only the starchy endosperm.

Why Brown Rice

- The fiber and phytonutrients in brown rice help lower cholesterol and prevent heart disease.
- Bran acts as a natural detoxifier that flushes out toxins.
- Fiber helps balance blood sugar levels.

Eat Brown Rice

- More than 8,000 varieties of rice and three basic types of rice – short, medium, and long grain – all available in their natural brown state.
- Flavorful basmati and jasmine.
- Chewy texture and hearty, nutty flavor.

2 Steel-Cut Oats: Ireland

Steel-cut oats are sometimes called Irish or Scottish oats and grow in the cold, wet climates of northern Europe and North America. Oats are unique among popular grains, as the bran and germ are rarely removed in processing.

Why Oats

- The fiber, beta-glucan, in oats helps lower cholesterol, which reduces the risk of heart disease and stroke, and enhances the body's immune system.
- Avenanthramide, a polyphenol antioxidant in oats, may have anti-inflammatory, heart-healthy, and anti-itch properties.
- Fiber helps us feel fuller longer, which controls weight.
- They have the highest protein content of popular cereals.

Eat Oats

- Available as steel-cut oats or oat groats (hulled grains).
- Do not eat instant quick-cooking oats. They are low in fiber because most of the bran is removed. In addition, sugars and preservatives are usually added to the package.
- The mild, smooth, sweet flavor makes oats a perfect breakfast grain to enjoy with nuts, seeds, and fruit.
- Oats are naturally gluten-free, but may be contaminated with gluten during growing and processing. Look for oats certified gluten-free if you are sensitive to gluten.

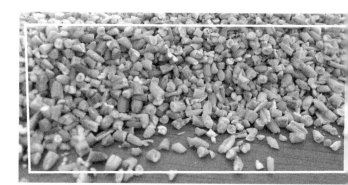

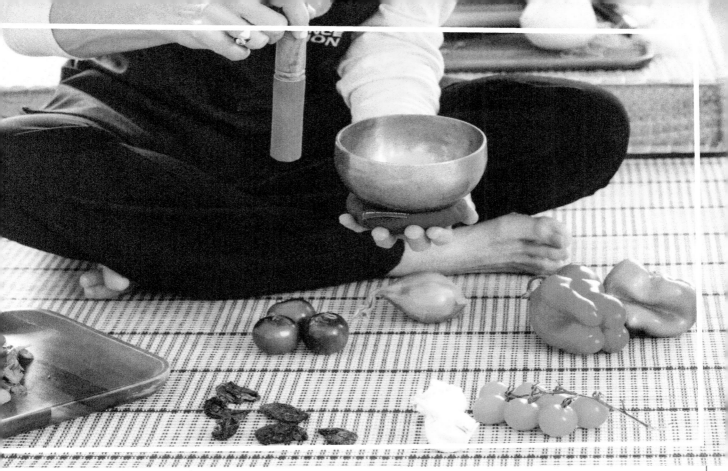

3 Spelt

Spelt is an ancient grain and a cousin of wheat that has been cultivated for 7,000 years. It was a staple in ancient Greece, ancient Rome, and medieval Europe. It has been grown in North America for just over 100 years.

Why Spelt

- Tough outer husk; because of this, requires less fertilizer and is more resistant to disease and pests
- Broader range of nutrients than wheat, including manganese, vitamin B2, niacin, thiamin and copper
- Fiber-rich, with 4 grams of fiber in one-half cup cooked spelt

" Celebrate the true beauty of food. **"**

Eat Spelt

- Because spelt contains less gluten than wheat, many people with gluten sensitivities can tolerate it. However, people with celiac disease should not eat spelt.
- Sweet and nutty; enjoy spelt cooked like brown rice.
- Enjoy making flatbread with sprouted spelt flour.

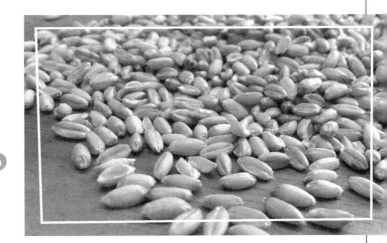

EXPLORE 4 PROTEIN-RICH GLUTEN-FREE PSEUDOGRAINS

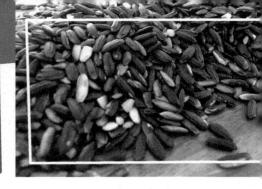

Grain-like foods – quinoa, kasha, wild rice, and amaranth – are really seeds that are naturally gluten-free and that contain more protein (20-25 percent) than whole grains.

1 Quinoa: Peru

Quinoa, the "mother of grains" as deemed by the Incans, was used as a chief source of nutrition for that civilization. Quinoa is actually the seeds of a plant related to chard and spinach.

Why Quinoa

- Protein-rich. Quinoa contains about 20 percent protein, twice the protein of rice.
- A complete protein. Contains all nine essential amino acids. It contains high levels of the amino acid lysine, essential for tissue growth and repair.
- Known to boost energy, help fight migraines and osteoporosis, and improve vision.

Eat Quinoa

- Versatile substitute for rice in a variety of colors: white, red, brown, pink, orange, and black.
- Fluffy, creamy, slightly crunchy texture, with a nutty flavor.
- Enjoy hot or cold. Cold salad or warm side dish with roasted veggies or wild salmon.

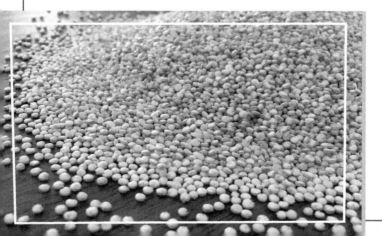

2 Wild Rice: Great Lakes

Wild rice is the seed of an aquatic grass originally grown by indigenous tribes around the Great Lakes. It now grows in Canada, Minnesota, and the Midwest.

Why Wild Rice

- Twice the protein and fiber of brown rice.

Eat Wild Rice

- Nutty, earthy taste and chewy texture.
- Often cooked with a blend of other grains.

> " If you are sensitive to gluten, do not eat it, as it can stay in your system for eight months. If you have celiac disease, you must go gluten-free. "

3 Buckwheat or Kasha: Russia

Buckwheat is popular in Eastern Europe and Asia. In Russia, it was often cooked for ceremonial meals like weddings and royal feasts. Buckwheat is a seed in the rhubarb family.

Why Kasha

- Almost a complete protein, as it contains eight amino acids.
- Nutrient-rich, with B vitamins, phosphorus, magnesium, iron, zinc, copper, and manganese. It's also a good source of an essential fatty acid known as alpha-linolenic acid.
- Fiber-rich, which helps control blood sugar and is beneficial for managing diabetes.
- Heart healthy. Rich in magnesium which lowers blood pressure. High in rutin, a flavonoid that improves circulation and prevents LDL (bad) cholesterol from blocking blood vessels.

Eat Kasha

- Sprouted buckwheat digests and burns efficiently.
- Popular in pancake mix, Japan's soba noodles, and Russia's kasha.
- Popular in cold weather. Enhance the hearty nutty flavor by pan toasting before cooking.
- Boil water before adding kasha to the pot.

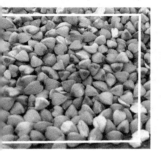 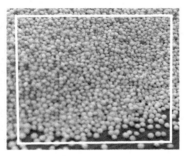

 # Amaranth: Mexico

Amaranth is a staple food of the Mexican Aztec culture; it is considered a native crop in Peru.

Why Amaranth

- A protein powerhouse; at 13-14 percent, it has a higher protein level than many grains.
- A complete protein because it contains lysine, an amino acid missing or negligible in many grains.
- Benefits heart health. Amaranth has shown potential as a cholesterol-lowering whole grain in several studies conducted over the past 14 years.

Eat Amaranth

- Nutty, crunchy, and peppery taste.
- Popular in cereals, breads, muffins, crackers, and pancakes. It can also be popped like popcorn.
- Cook with at least six cups of water for one cup of amaranth.

Get Clear on Gluten

Gluten is the protein in some grains that makes dough elastic. The primary grains with gluten include wheat, barley, rye, and triticale. The most popular wheat grains are bulgur, couscous, durum, faro, kamut, semolina, spelt, wheat berries, wheat bran, and wheat germ.

What is Gluten Sensitivity?

An estimated 15-35 percent of our population is sensitive to gluten, and many people have not been diagnosed. Gluten sensitivity causes inflammation in the body and could cause long-term damage such as intestinal scarring, nutrient malabsorption, and poor digestion.

Gluten sensitivity has widespread effects throughout the body:

- **Gut:** bloating, gas, acid reflux, indigestion, constipation, diarrhea, difficulty gaining weight, iron deficiency, anemia.
- **Head and nervous system:** headaches, sinus congestion, brain fog, ADD, ADHD, depression, anxiety, mood swings, MS or Parkinson's diagnosis, Alzheimer's.
- **Muscles and joints:** joint pain, muscle aches, muscle spasms, bone pain, growing pain, osteoporosis, fibromyalgia.
- **Hormonal:** fatigue, difficulty falling asleep, PMS, infertility, thyroid issues.
- **Immune problems**: asthma, infections.
- **Skin:** rash, hives, psoriasis.
- **Food cravings:** sweets.

Celiac Disease

Celiac disease is a lifelong digestive order that affects one out of every 133 people in the US. This number has increased four times over the last 50 years. The increase may be due to high levels of gluten and wheat in our diet. When we eat gluten (protein in wheat), it creates a toxic reaction from the immune system that causes damage to the small intestine, the loss of tiny villi which does not allow nutrients to absorb, and malnutrition.

Celiac disease is hard to diagnose, as it has either no symptoms or a variety of symptoms:

- Diarrhea
- Abdominal pain or bloating
- Weight loss
- Failure to grow (in children)
- Anemia
- Fatigue
- Malnutrition
- Osteoporosis
- Bone pain
- Depression

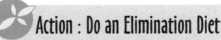 ## Action : Do an Elimination Diet

If you have several symptoms of gluten sensitivity, try an elimination diet. Do not eat gluten for two weeks; then add it back and notice how you feel. Do you have any of the gluten-sensitive symptoms? If you do have several symptoms, do a blood test or a stool and saliva test to test for gluten sensitivity.

4 WAYS TO PREPARE WHOLE GRAINS

In this section, you'll learn to cook grains for every meal:

- **Breakfast**: Steel-Cut Oats
- **Lunch:** Veggie Burgers
- **Dinner:** Pilaf and Risotto
- **Dessert:** Gluten-Free Apple Crisp

You'll learn how to prepare whole grains using four culinary methods to produce cuisine with different textures and flavors. These methods often require different types of grains.

1. **Steam:** Simple, basic way to cook whole grains in a rice cooker, on a stovetop, or in the oven.
2. **Pilaf:** Sauté grains in oil before adding liquid and be creative with extra vegetables, herbs, and spices.
3. **Risotto:** Slow, mindful cooking to bring out the starch in Arborio rice and create a creamy dish.
4. **Bake:** Cook grains in the oven for a veggie burger lunch or grain-based dessert.

Cooking Grains: How much and how long?

There are no absolute cooking times and liquid ratios when cooking grains. The amount of liquid and the cooking time depend on the type and age of the grains and the cooking method. For every 1 cup of whole grains, use the following guidelines.

Whole Grain	Liquid in Cups	Cooking Time Minutes
Amaranth	2-3	20-25
Brown rice	2-2.5	45-50
Kasha	1.5-2	20
Millet	1.5-2	25-30
Quinoa	1.75-2	15-20
Steel cut oats	2-2.5	20-30
Wild Rice	3	45-55

Get Clear on Rinsing and Soaking Grains

Rinse or Soak Grains?
Rinsing or soaking whole grains depends on whether or not the final dish is creamy.

- **Brown rice.** Soak long-grain brown rice to absorb water and reduce cooking time.
- **Basmati and jasmine rice**. Do not rinse, as the flavor of the rice is vital to the dish.
- **Pilaf.** Do not rinse or soak grains to be used in a pilaf, as the grains are first cooked with fat.
- **Arborio.** Do not soak Arborio, as the outer rice starch is vital to creating the creaminess in risotto.

How to Rinse Whole Grains
Rinse whole grains in cold water to remove the residue on the grains and as much of the outer starch as possible. If the excess starch is not removed, the grains become gummy. To properly rinse, place whole grains in a strainer in a bowl with running cold water. Agitate the grains with your hands and rinse several times until the water is clear.

How to Soak Whole Grains
Soak grains a few hours or overnight. Soaking grains allows the grains to absorb water, which allows the grains to cook more evenly and faster. After soaking, drain the grains well, as water absorbed in the grains may affect the ratio of water for cooking.

Simple Steps to Steam Perfect Whole Grains Every Time

The steaming method is a simple way to cook whole grains. With the steaming method, we use a specific amount of grain and a specific amount of liquid. We then cook for a specific amount of time. We can steam whole grains on the stovetop, in a rice cooker, or in an oven.

For all of these steaming methods the steps are: Rinse, add liquid, cover, cook, rest, fluff, rest, and serve.

8 Steps to Steam Grains on the Stovetop

By following the specific details in this step-by-step cooking process, you will cook perfect, flavorful, tender whole grains very time.

1. Rinse. Rinse whole grains to remove residue and extra outer starch.
2. Add liquid. Pour 1 cup of whole grains with 2 cups of water into a heavy pot. Use a heat diffuser under the pot to prevent the bottom layer of the grains from sticking.
3. Cover. Cover the pot and bring to a boil on medium-high heat.
4. Cook. Lower heat to lowest setting and simmer with the pot tightly covered for 15-20 minutes. Keep pot tightly covered to keep steam inside pot to cook the rice.
5. Rest the grains. Once cooked, remove the pot from the heat. For even cooking, uniform texture, and fluffier grains, rest the grains with the lid on the pot for 10-30 minutes.
6. Fluff the grains. Use a fork to lift the grains. Start at the bottom around the edge of the pot and lift the grains toward the center of the pot.
7. Rest. Cover and let the grains rest for another 10 minutes.
8. Serve. Plate and enjoy your perfect whole grains.

Steps to Steam Whole Grains in a Rice Cooker and Oven

- **Rice Cooker:** Pour rice and liquid into a rice cooker, cover, and turn on rice cooker. Let it cook. Rest. Fluff. Rest. Serve.
- **Oven:** After grains and liquid have come to a boil on the stove, cover and place in preheated 350-degree oven for 15-20 minutes. Cook. Rest. Fluff. Rest. Serve.

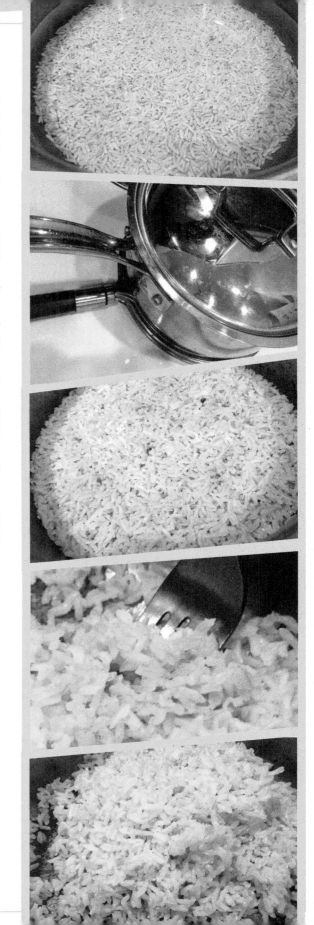

BREAKFAST WHOLE GRAINS: SIMPLE STEEL-CUT OATS IN RICE COOKER

Steel-cut oats make a quick, easy, and good-for-you breakfast. This recipe is the perfect foundation for a breakfast made with whole grains. You can use any whole grain and add your favorite nuts, seeds, trail mix, and fruit. The rice cooker method is a simple way to cook steel-cut oats as well as other whole grains.

SIMPLE INGREDIENTS

- 1 cup steel-cut oats
- ½ cup trail mix or your favorite nuts and seeds
- 2 ¼ cups water
- Organic apple, sliced
- Fresh grated cinnamon and nutmeg
- Local honey

SIMPLE STEPS

1. Thoroughly rinse steel-cut oats by placing them in a strainer and bowl of water. Rinse several times until the water is clear, not cloudy.
2. Pour steel-cut oats into a rice cooker.
3. Add trail mix, such as the EXPERIENCE NUTRITION Trail Mix, and sliced apple.
4. Pour water into the rice cooker.
5. Grate cinnamon and nutmeg into the rice cooker.
6. Turn on the rice cooker.
7. Oats will be ready when the cooker turns off, after about 20 minutes.
8. Enjoy with a drizzle of local honey.

Be Creative with Breakfast Whole Grains

Once you have made warm steel-cut oats, try other grains, such as quinoa, buckwheat (kasha), and even brown rice for breakfast. As with steel-cut oats, experiment with different extras, such as oranges and kumquats, pears, blueberries, raspberries, strawberries, and pomegranate seeds.

7 Culinary Tips to Make Whole Grains Even Better

1. **Buy bulk.** Typically, the best pricing and opportunity to try different whole grains.
2. **Grain liquid ratio.** Check information on the package or bulk section for ratios of grains to liquid. The ratio for brown rice and quinoa is approximately 1:2: 1 cup of grains to 2 cups liquid.
3. **Store in dark.** Store whole grains in a cool, dry, dark place in an air-tight container and use within six months. Glass jars work well.
4. **Add flavor.** To add interest to whole grains, add rough chopped fresh herbs, such as basil, cilantro, or lemon balm, or aromatics (finely chopped green onions) right before serving.
5. **Make a salad.** Toss cooked whole grains with fresh farmers' market veggies and a homemade lemon, olive oil, garlic dressing for a quick salad.
6. **Cool whole grains quickly, then refrigerate.** Spread whole grains on a flat baking sheet to cool, then cover and refrigerate. Eat cooked grains within two or three days.
7. **Warm pre-cooked whole grains.** Re-heat whole grains on stovetop or oven with a few tablespoons of added water to use in side dishes.

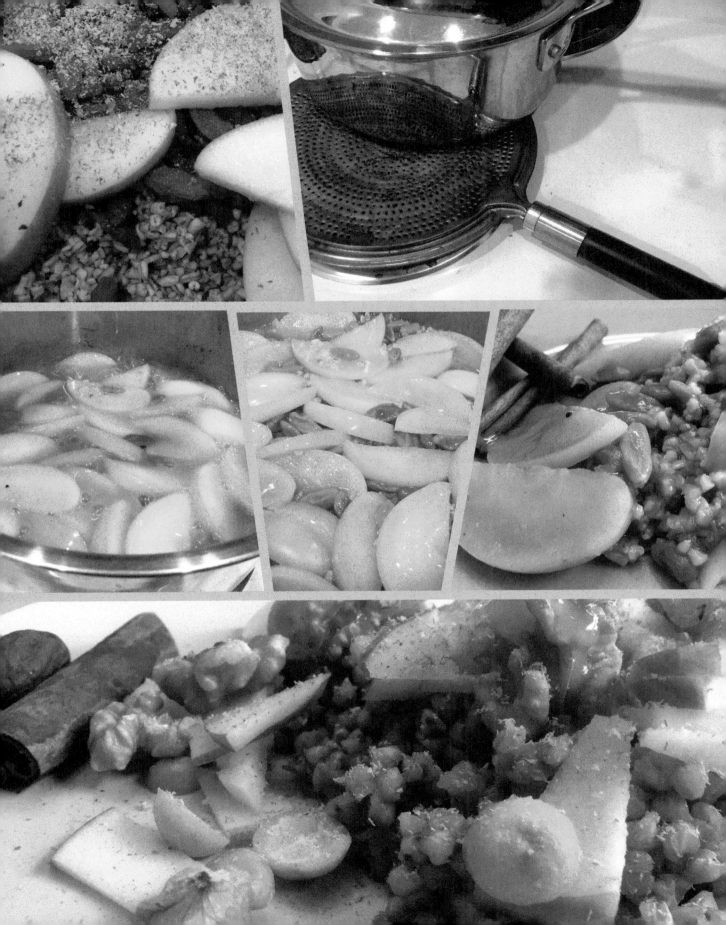

SIMPLE VEGGIE BURGER METHOD

LUNCH: Veggie Burgers

Veggie burgers are simple to make at home with whole grains, beans, veggies, fresh herbs, and spices. With this method of cooking, have fun experimenting with whole grains, cooked starchy vegetables, or beans as binders.

To create a wide variety of veggie burgers with different flavors, intuitively choose one item from each category and follow the simple steps to create tasty veggie burgers.

SIMPLE INGREDIENTS

Whole Grain: Cooked and cooled
- **Gluten-free:** Brown rice, quinoa, wild rice, amaranth, buckwheat, millet, oats
- **Gluten grains:** Wheat, barley, rye, bulgur

Plant Protein: Cooked legumes, nuts, or seeds
- Adzuki, cannellini, kidney beans, lentils, navy beans
- Almonds, cashews, walnuts, sunflower seeds

Vegetables: Raw, steamed, or roasted
- Broccoli, bell peppers, Brussels sprouts, cauliflower, celery, onions, snow peas, snap peas, tomatoes

Binder
- Whole grain cooked with extra water
- Cooked starchy vegetable: sweet potato, pumpkin, winter squash
- Beans, mashed
- Ground flax seeds or chia seeds with water (3:1 ratio of water:seeds)

Seasonings
- Fresh herbs: basil, cilantro, dill, lemon balm, mint, thyme
- Spices: garlic, ginger

Get to Know Different Types of Rice

Long-grain rice. Long and slender, holds its shape well, separates easily, and is light and fluffy when cooked. Long-grain rice works well in pilafs, soup, stir-fries, and salads. Popular long-grain rice varieties include basmati and jasmine. Basmati grows in the foothills of the Himalayas and has a fragrant, delicate flavor, as well as a long, slender shape. It is often cooked in Indian and Persian cuisine. Jasmine, originally from Southeast Asia (Thailand, Vietnam, and Cambodia), has a sweet, nutty flavor and aroma, and a soft, clingy texture.

Medium-grain rice. Shorter and wider than long-grain rice. When cooked, medium-grain rice is more moist and tender, and has a greater tendency to cling or stick together than does long-grain rice. Italian Arborio, with its high proportion of sticky starch, creates the creamy texture in risotto.

Short-grain rice. Almost round, short-grain rice has more starch than long-grain rice. Cooked short-grain rice is soft and tender, and clings or sticks together. Sushi rice is a popular short-grain rice.

SIMPLE STEPS

1. Preheat oven to 400 degrees F.
2. Combine whole grain, protein, and vegetables.
3. Add binder and mix until you can form a patty.
4. Season with herbs and spices.
5. Bake 10-12 minutes on parchment paper-lined flat baking sheet.
6. Flip patties.
7. Continue to bake 8-10 minutes or until center of the veggie burger is firm.
8. Enjoy.
9. Freeze leftovers with parchment paper between each veggie burger. Reheat in oven to enjoy later.

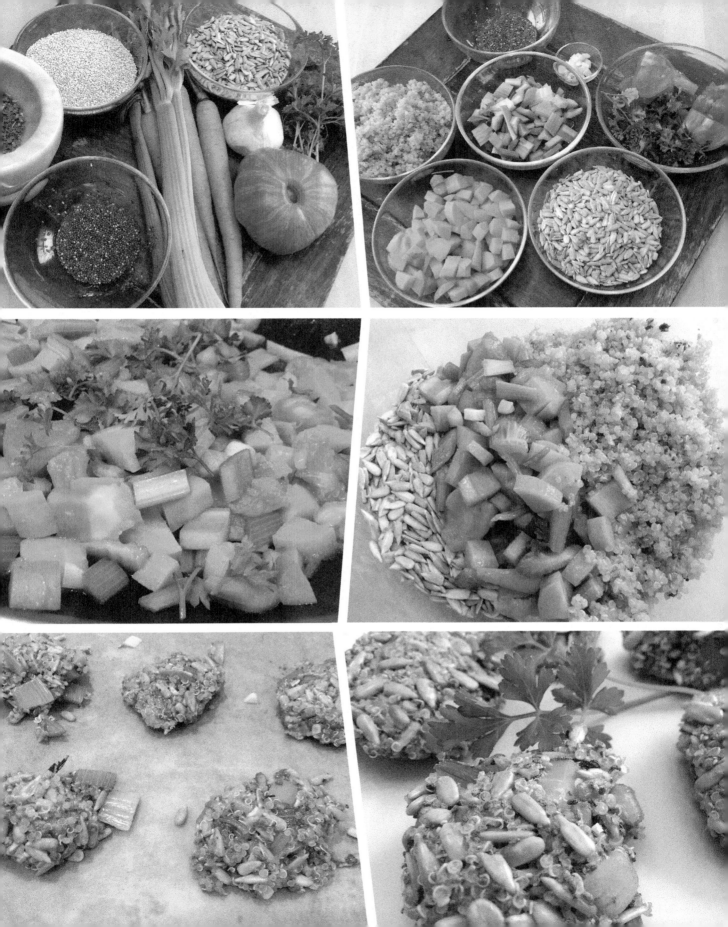

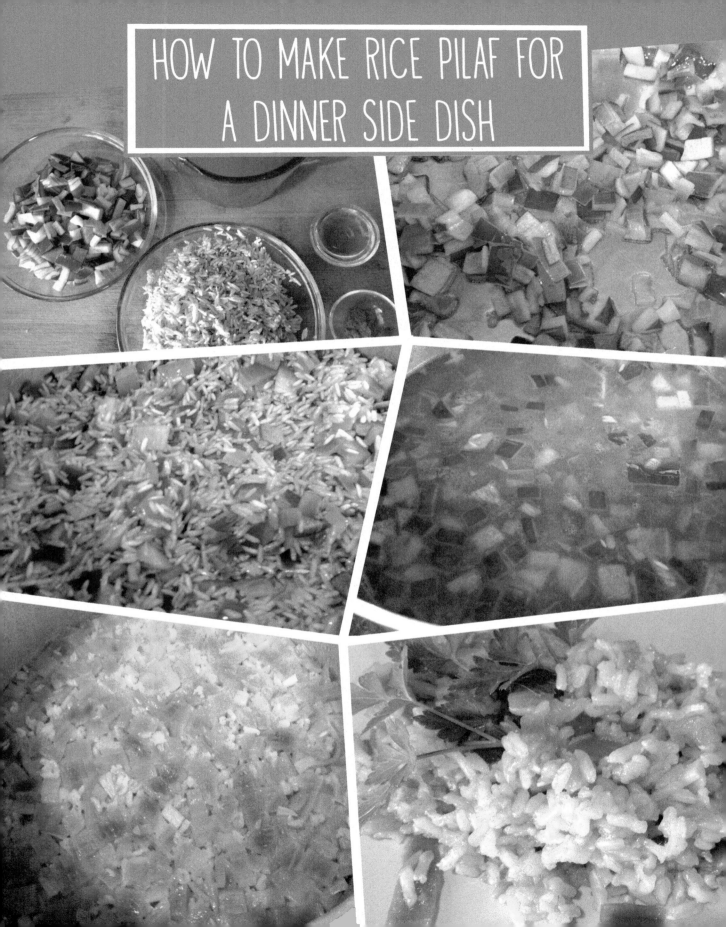

HOW TO MAKE RICE PILAF FOR A DINNER SIDE DISH

Pilaf is one of the main methods of cooking rice and is popular in Indian, Mexican, and Middle Eastern cuisines. The pilaf method is similar to steaming; however, in the pilaf method, whole grains are first sautéed, often with aromatics (like onions or shallots) before liquid is added, creating a lot of flavor. Pilafs also include extras such as vegetables and toasted nuts or seeds.

Simple Steps to Cook Using the Pilaf Method

1. In a sauté pan over low heat, cook mirepoix (carrots, onions, and celery or just onions) in a fat, such as olive oil. Cook on low heat when you do not want to add color to your dish. For more color, cook at a higher temperature.
2. Add grains to the pan and stir to lightly coat each grain with the fat. Do not rinse grains before cooking.
3. Toast grains by cooking a little more.
4. Add a flavorful liquid, such as vegetable stock.
5. Stir to make sure grain is not sticking to the bottom of the pan.
6. Similar to the whole grains steaming method, bring to boil, cover tightly, and reduce heat to the lowest setting (or cook in oven).
7. Cook a little longer than the time indicated for your grain and until all liquid is absorbed into the grains.
8. Rest grain for 10-20 minutes.
9. Fluff.
10. Rest for 10 minutes.
11. Serve.

Enhance Your Pilaf

To enhance the flavor and texture in your pilaf, add spices, herbs, fresh vegetables, nuts, and seeds.

- After the grains are coated in fat, add dried spices for extra flavor. Try Middle Eastern spices like star anise, cinnamon, and cumin. For a Mexican pilaf, add chili powder, cumin, cinnamon, and coriander seeds.
- After the cooked grains have rested, add your favorite cooked veggies, fresh herbs, or toasted nuts and seeds to create a meal.

Quick Brown Rice Turmeric Pilaf

SIMPLE INGREDIENTS

- 1 cup brown rice
- ¾ cup shallots or onions, finely diced
- 2-3 tbsp olive oil
- ½ tsp turmeric
- 2 cups vegetable stock

SIMPLE STEPS

1. Gather mise en place.
2. Sweat onions or shallots in olive oil.
3. Add rice and sauté until translucent.
4. Add turmeric for color.
5. Add vegetable stock.
6. Bring to boil.
7. Cover.
8. Cook for 20 minutes.
9. Rest for 10 minutes.
10. Fluff.
11. Serve.

DINNER: RISOTTO METHOD

Risotto is a beautiful, versatile, creamy Arborio rice dish. It's simple and mindful to prepare. Once you have mastered the risotto cooking technique, you can intuitively create delicious dishes with a variety of vegetables, sauces, oils, and fresh herbs. The key is to practice the risotto cooking technique and enjoy the mindfulness of the method, then cook your own versions of risotto.

I cooked my first risotto while studying with the Rouxbe Cooking School Plant-Based Professional Certification. I'm so glad I learned how to cook it. I often ordered risotto when eating out, and clearly recall a beautiful, delicious spring risotto with asparagus at one of my favorite vegan restaurants, Candle 79 in New York City. It was so delicious and creamy that I enjoyed it several weeks in a row when I was traveling to New York to study at the Institute for Integrative Nutrition.

Basic Risotto Cooking Method

SIMPLE INGREDIENTS

- 4-5 cups vegetable stock
- ½ cup onions, diced small
- ½ tsp sea salt
- 2 cloves garlic, finely minced, about the size of the rice
- 1 cup Arborio rice
- 2 tbsp extra virgin olive oil
- Optional: ¼ cup white wine
- Extras: Par-cooked vegetables such as carrots, green beans, peas, and asparagus

SIMPLE STEPS

1. Gather mise en place.
   - Vegetable stock, pre-heated on the stove
   - Onion and garlic, chopped
   - Rice, olive oil, sea salt (measured)
2. Start the risotto.
   - Place oil in a large, heavy-bottomed sauté pan and heat over medium-low heat.
   - Add onions and a pinch of salt. Sweat until soft and translucent, about 10-15 minutes.
   - Add ¼ cup of the hot cooking liquid (vegetable stock) to further soften the onions. Stir and cook until the liquid has completely evaporated.
3. Toast the rice and deglaze.
   - Turn heat to medium and add all the rice to the pan.
   - Stir constantly to coat rice in the hot oil.
   - Toast the rice for a few minutes until the edges of the grains are translucent.
   - Add the garlic and cook for 30 seconds to a minute.
   - Optional: Deglaze by stirring in wine until it evaporates.
4. Cook the risotto.
   - Risotto takes 20-30 minutes to cook. Start tasting for doneness at about 15 minutes.
   - Slowly add the hot liquid (vegetable stock) to the pan cup by cup and stir often to coax the starches out of the rice. Add the next cup of liquid after the previous liquid has completely absorbed. To test when to add more liquid, draw a track on the bottom of the pan as shown in the photo.
   - Adjust the heat so that the liquid is always gently boiling.
   - Continue to add the liquid until the rice reaches the al dente (almost tender) stage.
5. Finish the risotto
   - Stir in a little olive oil.
   - Optional: Fold in par-cooked vegetables.
   - Cover and rest for 1-2 minutes.
   - Just before serving, add a little hot liquid (vegetable stock) to loosen the consistency, if necessary.
   - Warm dishes in oven. Place dishes on a flat baking sheet and put in oven. Turn oven to its lowest setting (150 degrees F). Dishes will be warm in about 15 minutes.
   - Plate and drizzle with olive oil.
   - Serve immediately and enjoy.

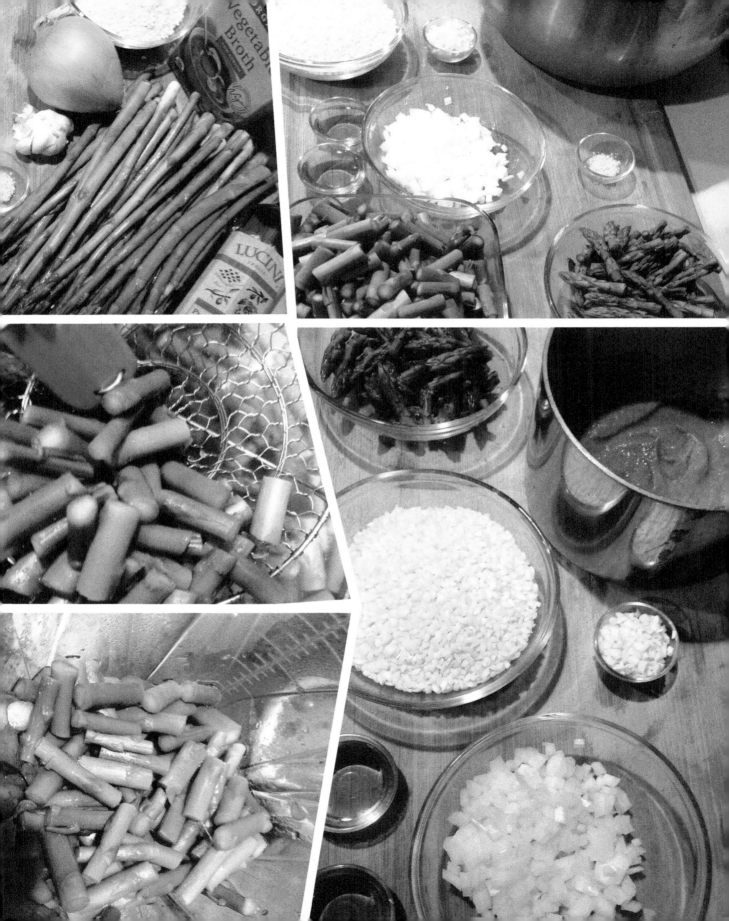

Culinary Tips to Make a Great Risotto

- **Arborio rice.** Italian grain. The starch in the rice creates the creamy sauce.
- **Do not rinse**. Never rinse the Arborio rice before cooking, as the outer starch is vital to making the creamy dish.
- **Basic ingredients.** 1 cup rice, 4-5 cups liquid, ½ cup mirepoix (onions, garlic), 2 tablespoons fat.
- **Heavy-bottom pan**. Use a heavy-bottom stainless steel, copper, or enamel cast iron pan for even heat distribution. Use a 3- to 4-quart pan with a depth of 2-3 inches.
- **Liquid options**. Use vegetable stock or broth. Because the stock will concentrate when cooked, use a liquid with a light flavor. Dilute the stock with extra water if desired. Season lightly with sea salt.
- **Add hot liquid while cooking**. Bring liquid (vegetable stock or broth) to boil in a separate pot, and heat on low to keep it hot during the cooking process, as the hot liquid helps release starch in the grain. Always have too much versus too little liquid available to use in your risotto.
- **Be mindful.** Notice how the starch from the rice creates a creamy texture and how the rice absorbs the vegetable stock or broth.
- **Experiment with vegetables.** Once you have practiced the risotto cooking method, experiment with different vegetables, such as farmers' market fresh carrots, beans, asparagus, or pea pods.
- **Finish risotto.** Try extra virgin olive oil, nut oils, pesto, or fresh herbs.

3 Beautiful Ways to Intuitively Create Unique Risotto

Once you have practiced the risotto cooking method, experiment with different sauces, vegetables, and finishes to intuitively create your own unique, tasty risotto dishes with different flavors and textures.

1. **Sauces.** 1 cup sauce (tomato) or vegetable puree (asparagus, butternut squash) for 1 cup dry rice. Use sauces with a pourable consistency. Warm sauce to simmer. Add sauce after the toasted rice has been deglazed. First, add 1 cup of the cooking liquid to the rice, then stir and cook until the liquid is absorbed into the rice. Next, add the heated sauce to the rice and simmer. Go back to adding additional cups of the cooking liquid, one by one, until the rice reaches al dente.

2. **Vegetables.** Try asparagus, carrots, beans, pea pods, fresh greens (spinach, arugula), or any combination of vegetables. Fold in par-cooked vegetables near the end of cooking (right before the rice rests) so that they do not overcook.

3. **Finishing.** Be creative with finishing with nut oils, pesto, and fresh herbs. Add these while plating the risotto.

❝ Cooking risotto is such a beautiful, mindful cooking process. I invite you to enjoy the process and share your risotto creations with us on www.facebook.com/NewViewHealthyEating. ❞

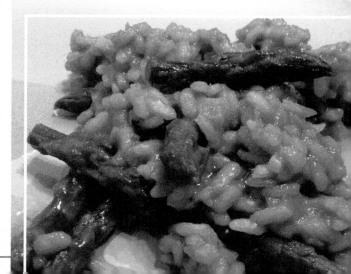

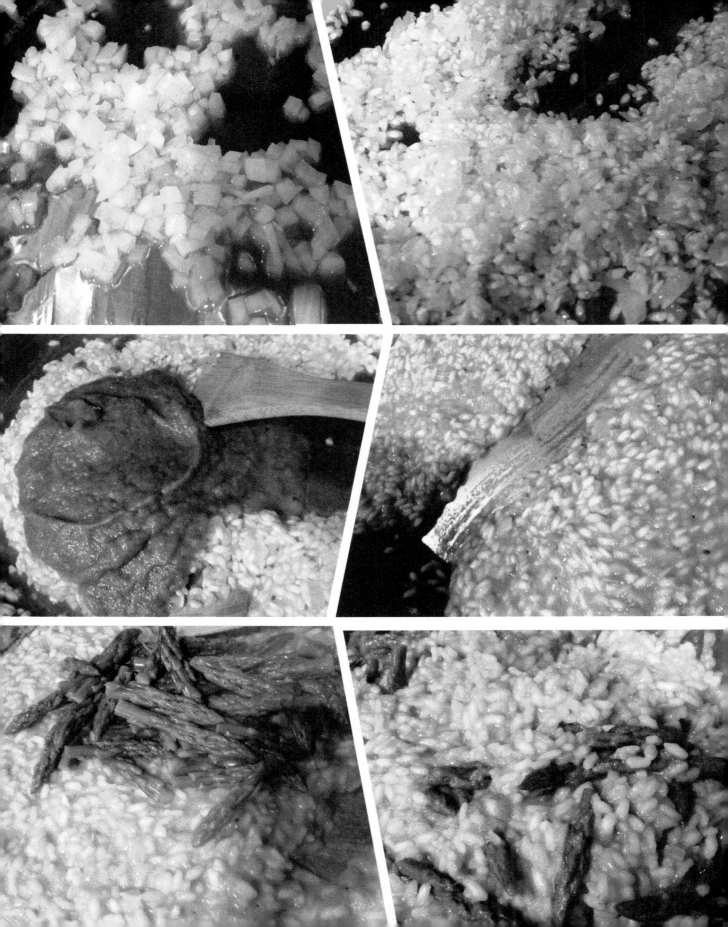

Have Fun with Simple Culinary Methods

I never imagined that I'd even try to make risotto and that it would taste so great when cooked at home. I totally enjoy the slow, mindful process of cooking risotto, and am always very proud of the beauty and delicious taste of the final dish. It is my pleasure to share the risotto cooking technique with those of you who, like me, have always wanted to cook risotto but never thought they would.

Experiment with Mirepoix

Mirepoix, the aromatic vegetables used at the beginning of the cooking process, builds the flavor profile of a dish. Different cuisines around the world typically begin their cooking with different combinations of vegetables. Experiment with various aromatic vegetables to create a wide variety of flavored dishes.

French: onions, celery, carrots
Italian: onions, celery, carrots, plus parsley, garlic, fennel
Mediterranean: onions, tomatoes, garlic, fennel
Spanish: onions, garlic, tomatoes
Asian: garlic, ginger, lemongrass
Cajun "Holy Trinity": onions, celery, green pepper
German: carrots, celery root, leeks

7 Simple Steps to Par-Cook Veggies

Par-cooking or par-boiling is used to partially cook vegetables for use in other dishes.

1. Bring a pot of cold water to a boil.
2. Season with salt.
3. Add the vegetables.
4. Cook vegetables to the almost al dente stage.
5. Shock in a bowl of water and ice to stop the cooking process and preserve color.
6. Once cooled, remove vegetables from the water.
7. Use the vegetables in risotto.

❝ Enjoy intuitively shopping at your local farmers' markets and then use your basic culinary skills to intuitively create simple, beautiful, tasty, healthy meals for you, your family, and friends. **❞**

3 Steps to Quickly Puree Vegetables

1. Simmer vegetables in a cooking liquid, such as vegetable stock, until tender.
2. Transfer to a blender with about ¼ cup of the cooking liquid and puree for at least 2 minutes until completely smooth.
3. Use the puree in risotto.

Action : Share Your Culinary Creations

Have fun in your kitchen with new culinary techniques and share your photos with us on Facebook: www.facebook.com/NewViewHealthyEating

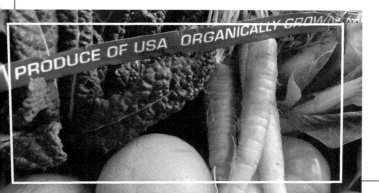

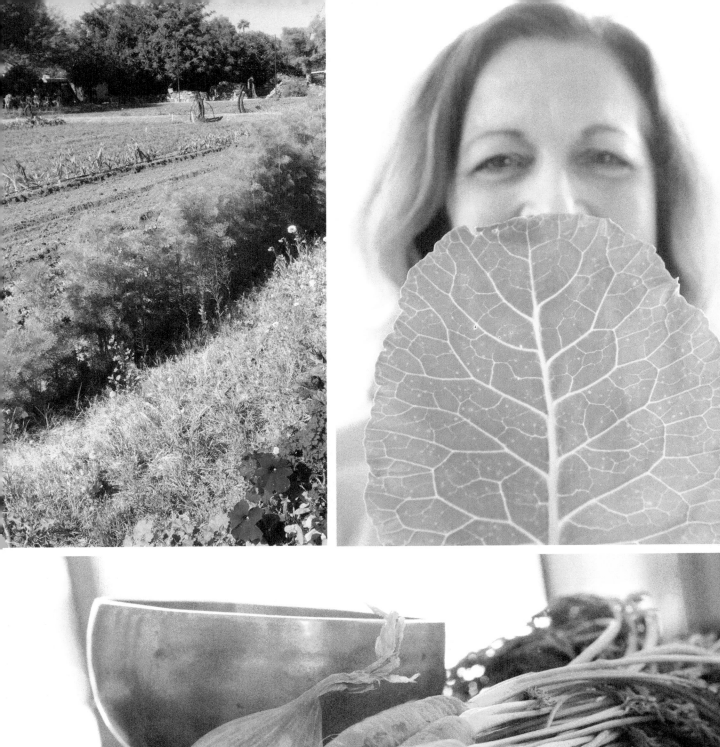
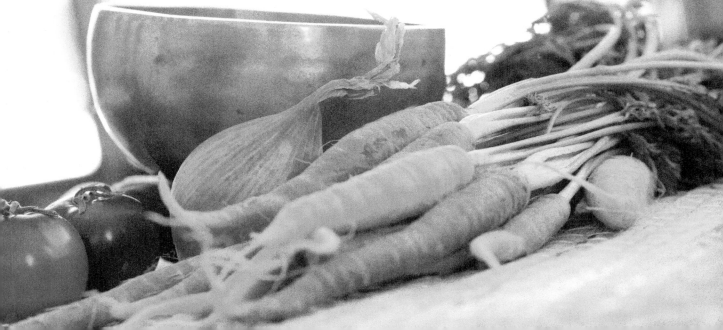

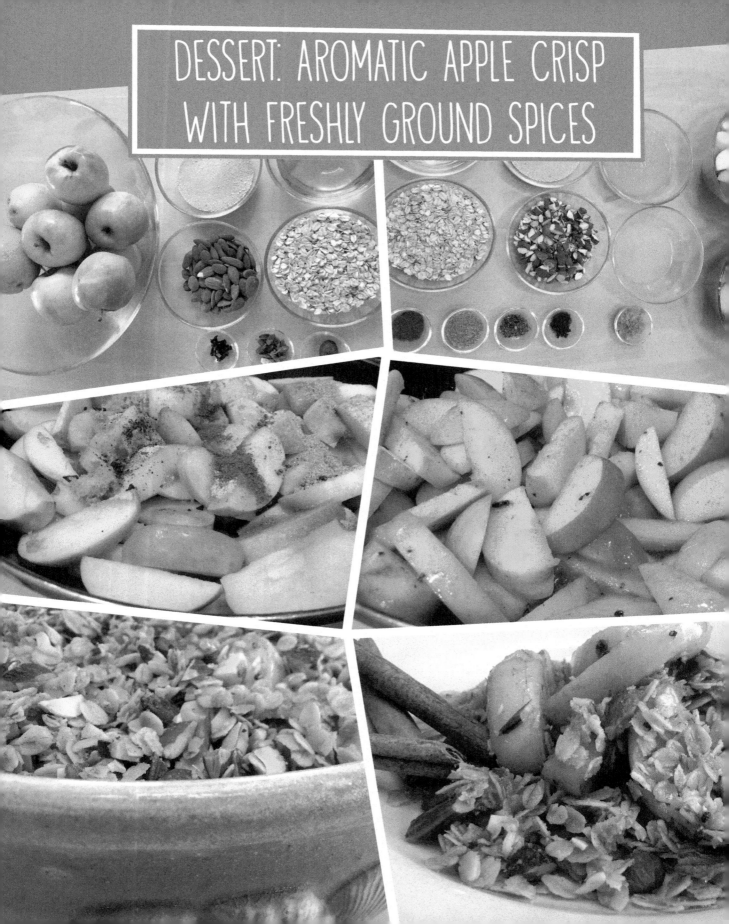

DESSERT: AROMATIC APPLE CRISP WITH FRESHLY GROUND SPICES

This apple crisp is one of my all-time favorites. From cooking with local organic apples to mindfully hand-grinding and enjoying the aromatherapy of freshly ground warming spices, from the aromatherapy of the apples sautéing in the spices to memories of eating pies when I was a child, this dessert (or breakfast) is outstanding. Enjoy the process of setting up your mise en place, cooking, and enjoying this dish with your family and friends.

SIMPLE INGREDIENTS

Topping

- 1 cup rolled oats
- ½ cup almonds, walnuts, or pecans, sliced
- ¼ cup maple sugar
- 1 tsp cinnamon, fresh ground
- 1 tsp nutmeg, fresh ground
- 1 tsp cardamom seeds, fresh ground
- ½ cup grapeseed oil

Filling

- 8 apples, sliced
- 3 tbsp grapeseed oil
- 4 tbsp maple sugar
- 1 tsp cinnamon, fresh ground
- 1 tsp nutmeg, fresh ground
- 1 tsp cardamom seeds, fresh ground
- ½ tsp cloves, fresh ground
- 1 orange, juiced and zested
- 1 lemon, juiced and zested

SIMPLE STEPS

1. Prepare your mise en place.
   - Hand-grind all spices in mortar and pestle.
   - Hand-squeeze and zest the orange and lemon.
2. Prepare topping.
   - Mix all dry ingredients for topping until well combined.
   - Pour in grapeseed oil and mix.
3. Cook the apple crisp.
   - Preheat oven to 350 degrees F.
   - Place sliced apples in a large sauté pan.
   - Turn heat to medium and add remaining filling ingredients.
   - Cook until apples slightly soften; stir occasionally.
   - Pour cooked apples with sauce into 8-inch by 8-inch baking dish.
   - Top with oats topping.
   - Bake on middle oven rack for 20-30 minutes.
4. Enjoy!

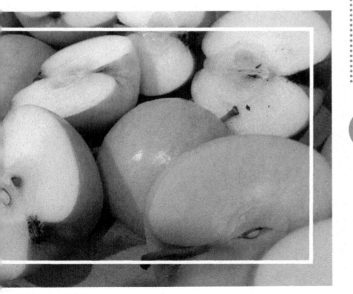

Action : Experiment with Whole Grains

In this section we've explored several ways to cook and enjoy whole grains: steaming on the stove or rice cooker for a quick breakfast, making pilaf for a side dish, creating a variety of veggie burgers, cooking a beautiful risotto, and preparing a naturally aromatic apple dessert. I invite you to experiment with two culinary methods of preparing whole grains. First, learn the method, then use your intuition when shopping and planning your meal to create your own delicious, beautiful, grain-rich dishes.

Cook and Eat Wild Salmon at Home

Culinary
- Simple way to grill and broil salmon
- Make your own salmon marinate
- Learn to poach salmon
- Top 4 tips to shop for fish

Recipes
- Wild Alaskan Sockeye Salmon on the Grill
- Wild Alaskan Sockeye Salmon Salad
- Simple Poached Salmon

Nutrition
- Get clear on omega-3 essential fatty acids OR Why we must eat omega-3 fatty acids
- EPA and DHA essential fatty acids in fish
- Top omega-3 rich fish
- How to balance omega-6s with omega-3s

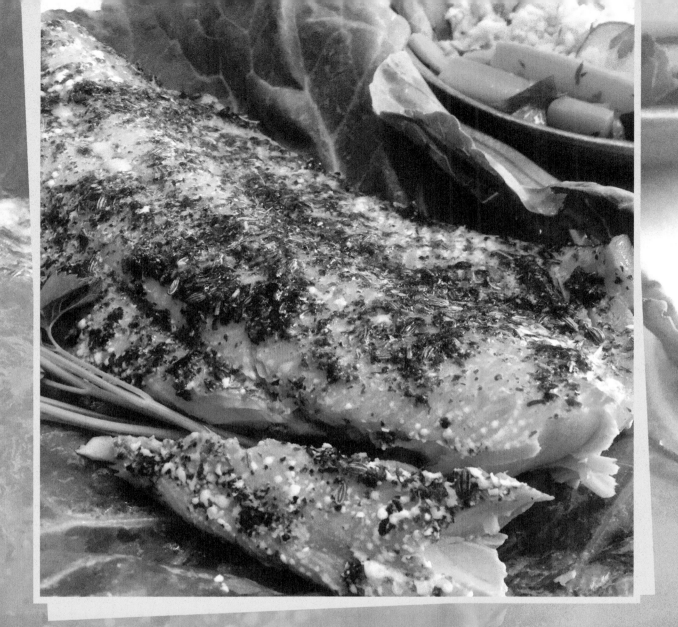

COOK AND EAT WILD
SALMON AT HOME

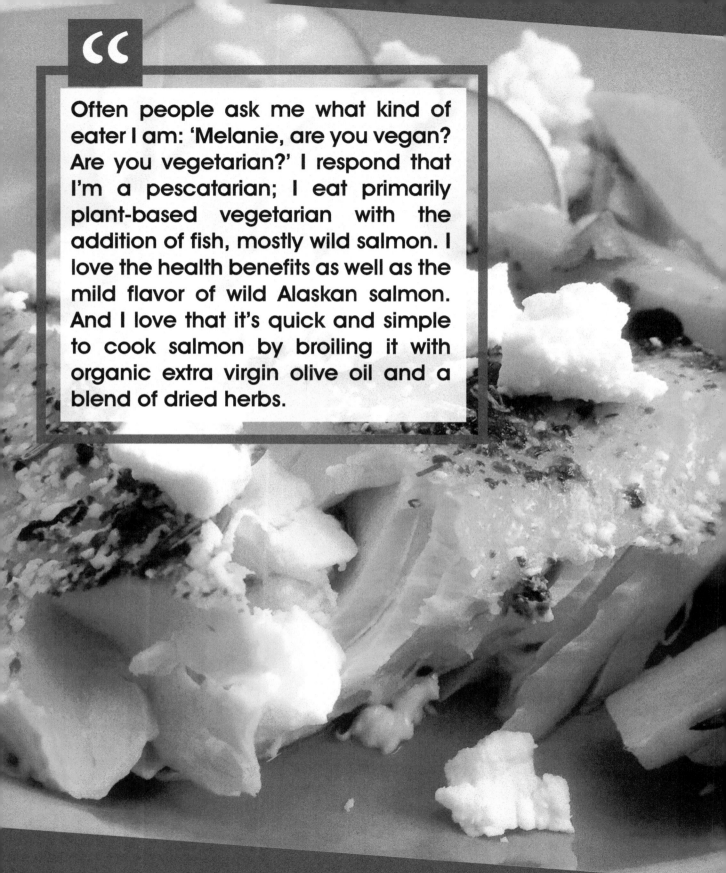

Often people ask me what kind of eater I am: 'Melanie, are you vegan? Are you vegetarian?' I respond that I'm a pescatarian; I eat primarily plant-based vegetarian with the addition of fish, mostly wild salmon. I love the health benefits as well as the mild flavor of wild Alaskan salmon. And I love that it's quick and simple to cook salmon by broiling it with organic extra virgin olive oil and a blend of dried herbs.

Eat Wild Salmon

Salmon contains powerful omega-3 essential fatty acids, which are anti-inflammatory and protective for heart health, brain health, diabetes, and joint pain. Often we eat salmon only when dining out. In this section, you'll learn simple ways to cook delicious wild salmon right in your home.

It has been such an honor to share with many people the value of eating omega-3-rich salmon and, importantly, simple ways to prepare it. I have shared this information with:

- MDs and healthcare professionals at the Marquette General Hospital 2011 Nutrition & Medicine Conference
- Former NFL players in their homes, including Super Bowl champion Seth Joyner, veteran quarterback Dave Krieg, former Arizona Cardinal John Bronson, and NFL wife Ericka Lassiter.
- Former NFL players at several NFL Alumni Association events during the 2011 Super Bowl XLV week in Dallas.
- People with Parkinson and their families at the 2015 Parkinson Wellness Recovery Retreat in Scottsdale.
- Men of the Mankind Project while catering a 2015 retreat weekend in Tempe, Arizona.

To get clear on why omega-3-rich cold-water fatty fish like wild salmon is vital for health, we will explore:

- The benefits of eating foods rich in omega-3 essential fatty acids
- Top omega-3-rich fish
- How to shop for fish
- Why to eat wild versus farmed fish
- How to balance omega-6s with omega-3s

In this section, you'll learn three simple ways to prepare fish so that you'll be comfortable cooking at home for your family and friends. You'll learn how to:

- Cook salmon on the grill or in the broiler
- Create a salmon salad in minutes
- Poach flavorful, mouthwatering salmon with fresh lemon and herbs

Melanie grilling salmon with former NFL player, John Bronson.

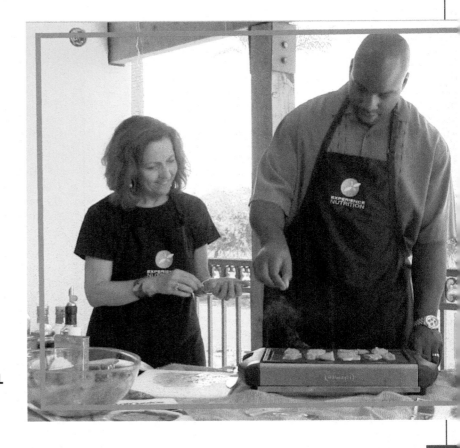

WILD ALASKAN SOCKEYE SALMON ON THE GRILL

Wild salmon is a rich source of anti-inflammatory omega-3 fatty acids, a good source of protein, and rich in Vitamin D, which is important for bone health, the immune system, and brain health.

In 2011, as an Official Health & Wellness Partner of the NFL Association, my organization Experience Nutrition Group, LLC had the honor of serving this simple Wild Alaskan Salmon recipe at several Super Bowl XLV weekend events in Dallas. Former NFL players kept coming back for more salmon, so apparently they enjoyed it. The recipe is very easy to prepare and delicious every time. Grill or broil the wild salmon with a few spices and olive oil to create a restaurant-quality meal quickly in your home.

Grill or broil wild Alaskan salmon using this simple recipe as a guide. Then, be creative and intuitively prepare the salmon with your favorite dried spices and herbs.

SIMPLE INGREDIENTS

- 4 wild Alaskan sockeye salmon fillets (4-6 oz. per person), sliced into ½-inch strips
- ¼ cup organic extra virgin olive oil
- 3 tbsp dried herbs and spices

Make Your Own Salmon Marinate

Create a total of 3 tablespoons of dried spices and herbs. Try a mix of garlic granules, onion granules, dried dill, lemon peel, fennel, black pepper, and sea salt. Or, experiment with dried basil, marjoram, oregano, and sea salt. Hand-grind the spices and herbs in a mortar and pestle and then mix with ¼ cup of olive oil to create your salmon marinade.

SIMPLE STEPS

1. Defrost salmon fillets in a refrigerator for a few hours or under cold running water.
2. Slice wild salmon into thin strips, about ½ inch wide and 1-2 inches long.
3. Prepare salmon marinade by mixing olive oil and spices and herbs.
4. Marinate salmon with spices and herbs in a refrigerator for 20-30 minutes, or overnight.
5. Pre-heat grill on medium high for 15 minutes before you are ready to cook the salmon. If broiling, preheat broiler for 15 minutes.
6. Place fillets directly on the grill or on a flat baking sheet with parchment paper for broiling.
7. Cook each side 3-5 minutes.
8. Remove salmon from grill right before it has completely cooked, as it will continue to cook when removed from the heat of the grill.
9. Let salmon rest for 5 minutes.
10. Enjoy with a veggie stir-fry, steamed vegetables, or a raw kale salad, with a side of whole grains such as quinoa or brown rice.

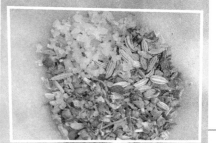
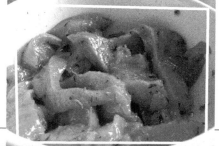
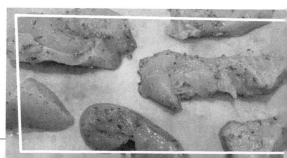

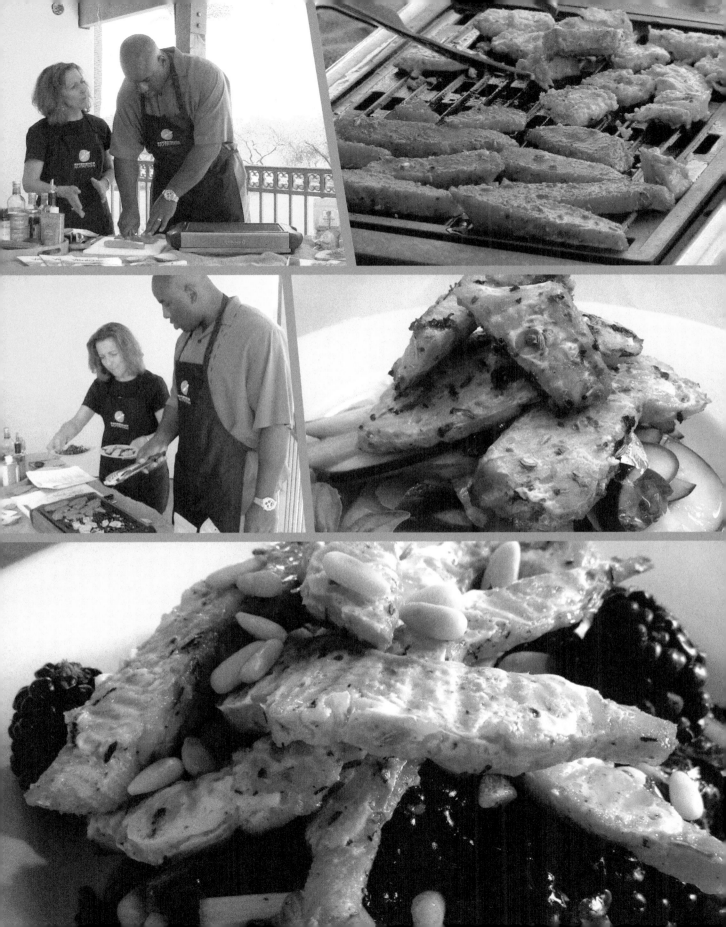

Why We Must Eat Omega-3s

For optimal health, we must eat about 30% good fats every day, every meal. Omega-3 fatty acids are important for many areas of health, including:

- Reduce inflammation, which is often considered the root cause of many diseases, such as heart disease, many cancers, and Alzheimer's disease
- Lower risk of heart disease: lower blood pressure, triglycerides (blood fat), and cholesterol
- Improve brain health, which positively influences memory
- Help depression and mental health, and may be beneficial for ADHD, autism, and dementia
- Reduce joint inflammation and pain
- Reduce risk of diabetes
- Benefit bone health
- Protect eye health
- Synthesize hormones
- Reduce risk of cancer

Omega-3 fatty acids are found in beef, eggs, and poultry, but are most abundant in the fat of cold-water, oily fish. Omega-3 fatty acids are also available in supplement form.

EPA and DHA Essential Fatty Acids in Cold-Water Fish

Cold-water fatty fish are a rich source of the two essential omega-3 fatty acids: EPA (eicosapentaenoic acid) and DHA (docosahexaenoic acid). These nutrients benefit long-term physical and mental health. EPA supports heart health, and DHA supports brain development and function.

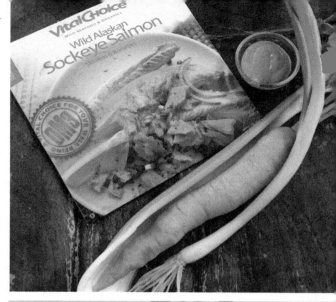

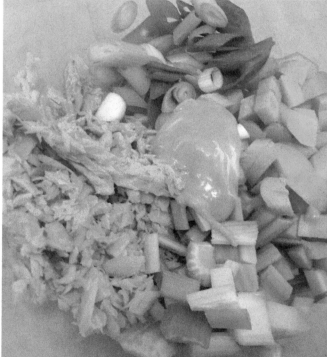

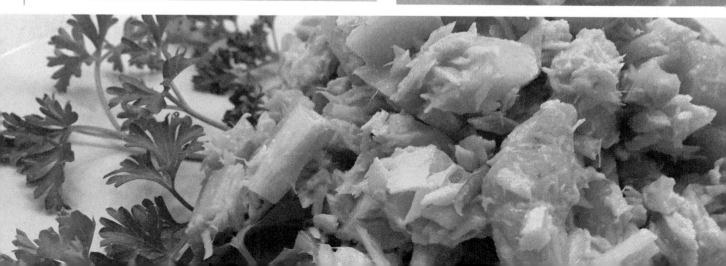

Wild Alaskan Sockeye Salmon Salad

In the summer of 2015, I had the opportunity to lead the creation of this salmon salad at the Parkinson Wellness Recovery Retreat for 168 people. I honestly think that everyone in the two weekends of the retreat absolutely loved the simplicity of preparing this salad and its refreshing taste. Some of my cooking friends and I also created this salmon salad recipe for catering at a weekend retreat with the non-profit ManKind Project, which also loved the salad.

For a simple, delicious alternative to tuna, try wild Alaskan sockeye salmon with fresh veggies to create a simple omega-3-rich salad. You can choose salmon with or without skin and bones.

SIMPLE INGREDIENTS

- 6-oz. can wild Alaskan sockeye salmon
- 2 tbsp stone ground or Dijon mustard
- 1 celery stalk, minced
- 1 green onion, diced
- 1-2 rainbow carrots, sliced
- Black pepper, to taste

SIMPLE STEPS

1. Chop celery, onions, and carrots.
2. Gently mix all ingredients.
3. Enjoy on top of a simple raw kale salad: kale, organic extra virgin olive oil, lemon juice, fresh garlic, and sea salt.

Top 4 Tips to Shop for Fish

1. **Eat Smaller Fish such as Salmon, Sardines, and Mackerel**
   - Smaller fish are lower on the food chain, and, therefore, contain fewer toxins, mercury, and contaminants from pollution in lakes, rivers, and oceans.
   - Do not eat predatory fish like swordfish, marlin, and shark, which have high levels of toxins (mercury and PCBs).
   - Avoid tilapia, as it is mostly farmed.

2. **Buy Wild, Not Farmed, Fish**
   - Wild cold-water fish have higher levels of beneficial omega-3 fatty acids.
   - Wild sockeye salmon eat a natural diet of krill (small crustaceans) and phytoplankton (microalgae) as opposed to fish, so they have the most astaxanthin (a powerful antioxidant) and obtain a deeper orange hue than other species.
   - Sockeye salmon cannot be farm-raised.

3. **Do Not Eat Farmed Salmon**
   - It contains a higher ratio of pro-inflammatory omega-6s to anti-inflammatory omega-3s.
   - It has less protein and flavor.
   - It contains residues of pesticides, antibiotics, and other drugs used to control diseases that occur when fish are crowded together in the pens of fish farms.
   - It is fed food pellets to grow and produce its orange color. Food pellets are made of meat and bone meal from the leftover meat, blood, and bones of animals, as well as larger fish that contain PCBs.

4. **Buy Sustainable Fish for the Environment**
   - It is estimated that 75% of the world's fisheries are fished to capacity or overfished.
   - Look for the Marine Stewardship Council Certified Sustainable Seafood label, which indicates that the fish were caught or raised in a sustainable, environmentally friendly manner.

SIMPLE POACHED WILD SALMON

Enjoy rich, flavorful poached wild salmon with fresh lemon juice and herbs.

SIMPLE INGREDIENTS

- 4 6-oz. wild salmon filets
- 3-4 carrots, sliced
- 1 small onion, sliced
- 3-4 celery stalks, sliced
- 4 slices fresh lemon
- ½ lemon, juiced
- Several sprigs of parsley and/or dill

SIMPLE STEPS

1. Cut salmon fillets into individual portions, if necessary.
2. Place carrots, onion, celery, lemon slices, lemon juice, and fresh parsley and/or dill into a small pot.
3. Add salmon to the pot, then add cold water to cover all ingredients.
4. Bring the water to a boil.
5. Uncover the pot.
6. Lower heat to simmer and cook for about 5 minutes.
7. Turn off heat and let salmon continue to cook in the liquid for 10 minutes.
8. Carefully remove salmon from the pot and serve.
9. Enjoy hot or cold.

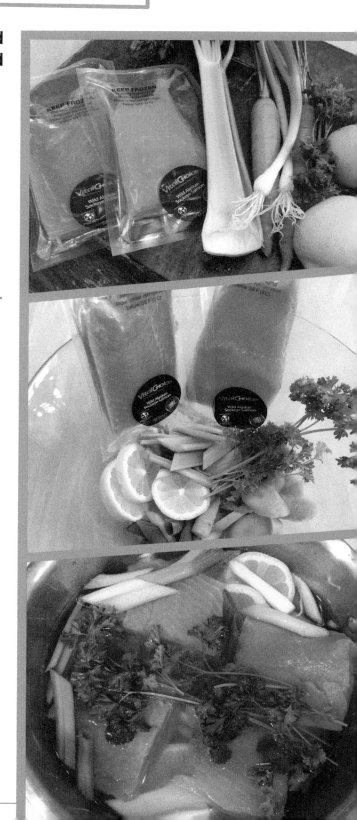

Huge Omega-3 and Omega-6 Imbalance in the US Today

Until about 50 years ago, our diets contained about 3 parts omega-6s to 1 part omega-3s. Today, the average American eats too many pro-inflammatory omega-6s and not enough omega-3s. The American diet contains about 20 to 40 times as much omega-6s as omega-3s due to the enormous increase of omega-6s in our food today.

Stop Eating Omega-6 Fats

- Omega-6s are pro-inflammatory and found in vegetable oils such as corn, soybean, sunflower, and safflower oil. These omega-6 fatty acids are ingredients in many processed foods and are used in cooking in most restaurants and homes across the US.

- The imbalance of omega-6s to omega-3s promotes heart disease, cancer, diabetes, and dementia.

- The ideal ratio of omega-6s to omega-3s is 2:1 to 4:1. That is we should be eating only two to four times as much omega-6s as omega-3s, as compared to the 20 to 40 times as much in the typical US diet.

How Much Omega-3-Rich Food Do You Need to Eat?

To help get our omega-3 and omega-6 ratio at a more healthy level, the amount of omega-3s we need to eat depends on each of our individual eating habits and preferences.

Standard American Diet Eater

If you eat the typical Standard American Diet (SAD), you need to eat more omega-3s. Eat 6 ounces of wild omega-3-rich fish every day. The SAD way of eating includes high levels of omega-6s, a lot of processed foods, restaurant dining, and large amounts of meat, poultry, eggs, and dairy. A landmark study showed that most Americans need to eat 3.5 grams omega-3-rich (EPA and DHA) fish a day to match Japan's low rates of heart disease and depression.

Eat Good Plant Fats and Cook at Home Eater

If you eat healthy plant fats (like extra virgin olive oil, avocados, nuts, and seeds), cook whole food meals at home, and do not typically eat processed foods, you do not need to eat as many omega-3s. Eat three or four servings weekly of omega-3-rich fish such as wild salmon, or take fish oil supplements.

Top Omega-3-Rich Fish

Omega-3s: mg per 3 oz. serving	
Pacific Herring (Sardines)	1,604
Black Cod	1,410
European Anchovies	1,256
Spanish Mackerel	1,255
Wild Sockeye Salmon	948

Action : Experiment with wild cold-water fish.

In this section, we've explored several ways to cook and enjoy wild salmon: grilling, as a salad, and poached. If you are a fish eater, I invite you to experiment with one culinary method of preparing wild salmon. Shop for an omega-3-rich wild salmon and cook it for your family or friends.

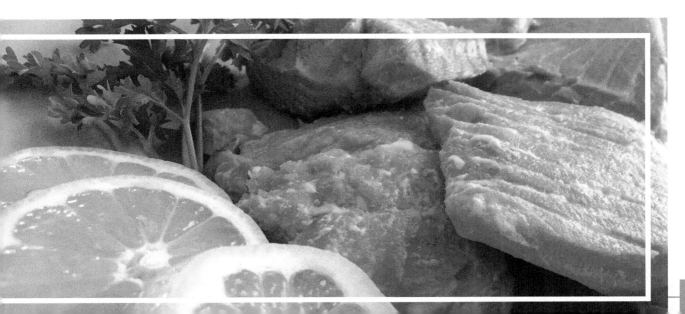

Get Creative with Nuts and Seeds

Culinary

- 5 tips to shop for and enjoy nuts and seeds
- 5 simple steps to make your own nut and seed milk
- 6 nuts and seed milk tips
- Quick and easy steps to make your own raw nut butter
- How to make raw nut and seed pates
- Top 5 ways to enjoy seeds every day
- 5 ingredients for dehydrated flatbread

Recipes

- Pomegranate Smoothie with Homemade Almond Milk
- Simple Raw Almond Butter
- Basic Almond Pate
- Mediterranean Almond Pate with Organic Heirloom Tomatoes, Kalamata Olives, and Capers
- Pecan Pate with Red Peppers and Ginger
- Raw Taco Salad
- Hemp Seed Tabouli with Heirloom Tomatoes
- Sweet Pepper Almond Flaxseed Raw Dehydrated Crackers

Nutrition

- Why nuts and seeds are good for us
- The fats in nuts and seeds
- Protein in nuts and seeds
- Get clear on plant-based omega-3s
- Why eat hemp seeds

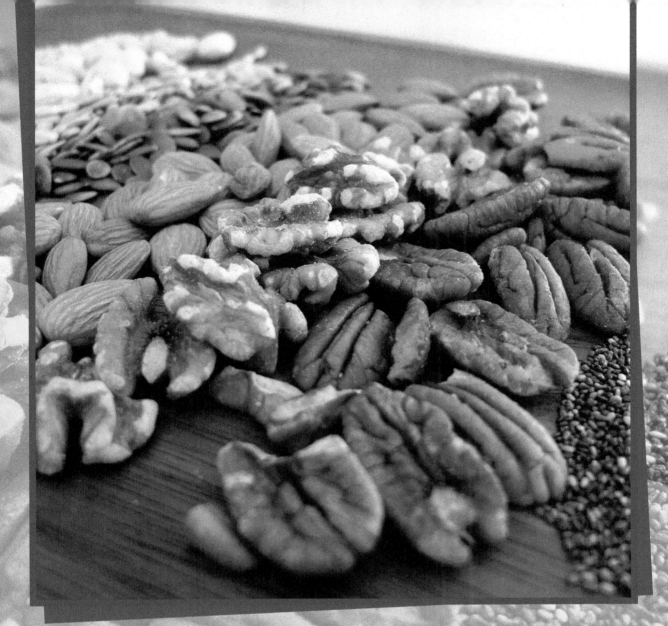

GET CREATIVE WITH
NUTS AND SEEDS

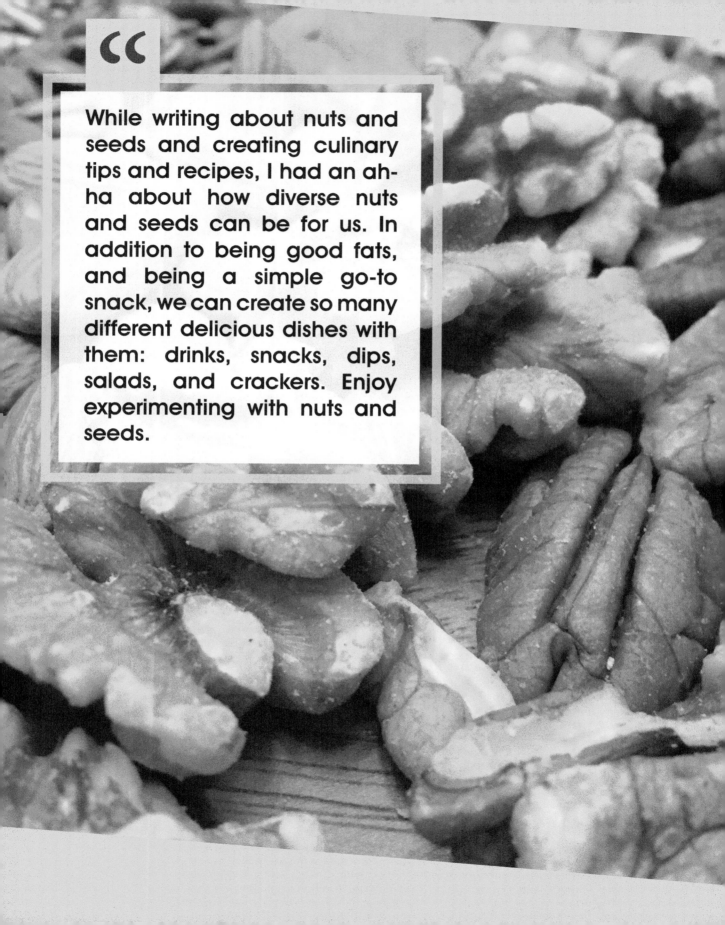

" "

While writing about nuts and seeds and creating culinary tips and recipes, I had an ah-ha about how diverse nuts and seeds can be for us. In addition to being good fats, and being a simple go-to snack, we can create so many different delicious dishes with them: drinks, snacks, dips, salads, and crackers. Enjoy experimenting with nuts and seeds.

GET CREATIVE WITH NUTS AND SEEDS

Nuts and seeds are good fats

For decades, many people stayed away from eating nuts and seeds because they are full of fat. The media told us that fats cause fat, and there have been many popular low-fat diets over the years. Today, we do see in the news that we can eat fat, but many people are still confused about which foods contain healthy fats.

To get clear on why we can eat fat-rich nuts and seeds, we will explore:

- Why nuts and seeds are good for us
- The fats in nuts and seeds
- Hemp seeds, which are a complete protein

Many people eat nuts and seeds as a snack. In this section, you'll learn several great ways to enjoy nuts and seeds, in addition to eating them by the handful. You'll learn how to create:

- Your own nut and seed milk
- Homemade raw nut butter
- Raw nut and seed pâtés: almond, walnut, Mediterranean, and raw taco salad
- Hemp seed tabouli with heirloom tomatoes
- Dehydrated raw flaxseed crackers

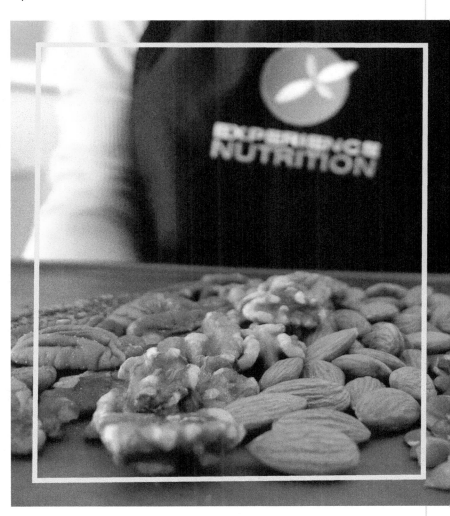

GET TO KNOW THE FATS IN NUTS AND SEEDS

One way to think about nuts and seeds is that they are the fat that grows on plants. Nuts and seeds contain 65-85% fat and are comprised of different types of fats, including monounsaturated, saturated, and polyunsaturated fats (omega-3 and omega-6).

Most of the fat in many nuts and seeds is monounsaturated and good for the heart. Nuts and seeds are generally rich in vitamin E, trace minerals, and fiber. Sunflower and pumpkin seeds contain both polyunsaturated and monounsaturated fats. Walnuts and pine nuts are rich in polyunsaturated fats. Chia seeds, hemp seeds, and flaxseeds are very rich in heart-healthy omega-3 fatty acids.

Monounsaturated Rich: Macadamia, cashews, hazelnuts, pecans, almonds

Monounsaturated/Polyunsaturated Rich: Sunflower seeds, pumpkin seeds

Polyunsaturated Rich: Walnuts, pine nuts

Omega-3-Rich Seeds: Flax seeds, chia seeds, hemp seeds (also a complete protein)

Protein-Rich Nuts and Seeds

In addition to being rich in good-for-us fats, nuts and seeds are an excellent source of protein for those who eat a plant-based diet. Because of their high protein levels, nuts and seeds satisfy appetites, control cravings, and help with weight management. Their high protein levels make nuts and seeds a great snack for an energy boost.

% Protein in Nuts & Seeds

Hemp seeds	33
Pumpkin seeds	21
Sunflower seeds	17
Black walnuts	13
Pistachios	13
Sesame seeds	13
Almonds	12
Cashews	12
Flaxseeds	12
Chia seeds	11
Hazelnuts	8
Walnuts	8
Pecans	5

Fat Composition of Nuts and Seeds

% Fat	MUFA	PUFA	SFA	Grams of fat per 1 cup
Macadamia	88	78.9	2.0	16.2
Cashews	66	53.6	17.6	17.6
Hazelnuts	81	52.5	9.1	5.1
Pecans	87	44.5	23.6	6.7
Almonds	72	29.3	11.5	3.5
Sunflower seeds	74	25.9	32.4	6.2
Pumpkin seeds	71	19.7	28.8	12.0
Pine nuts	85	25.3	46.0	6.6
Walnuts	83	10.5	55.2	7.2

Key: MUFA (Monounsaturated Fatty Acid), PUFA (Polyunsaturated Fatty Acid), SFA (Saturated Fatty Acid)

Source: Compiled from SELFNutritionData.com

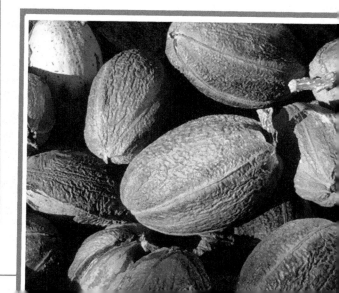

Make Your Own Nut or Seed Milk

Nut milks are very popular, but often store-bought milks contain added sugars or preservatives. Use these simple steps to make your own nut milks, which are nutrient-dense, more affordable than store-bought milks, and taste so fresh. Enjoy your made-from-scratch nut milk as a beverage, in smoothies, or in recipes that call for milk.

When making nut milk, it's important to remember that various nuts and seeds have different flavor profiles, from neutral, to slightly sweet, to slightly bitter. Intuitively create your own favorite nut milk by experimenting with different nuts and seeds.

- **Neutral:** Almonds, Brazil nuts
- **Slightly sweet:** Cashews, macadamia, pecans
- **Slightly bitter, may need to balance with a sweetener:** Seeds

Nut-Based Milk. Generally, nut milk, such as almond, tends to be white and watery, with a thin texture and a mild, almost bland flavor. Use almond milk as a great plant-based replacement for milk or water in smoothies or with morning whole grains, such as steel-cut oats.

Seed-Based Milk. Seed milk, such as hemp milk, is thick and creamy. Hemp milk made with dates and vanilla has a lot of depth and a flavorful, sweet, nutty, earthy taste. Drink hemp milk as a perfect healthy beverage.

5 Simple Steps to Make Your Own Nut or Seed Milk

1. Pour $1/3$ cup raw nuts or seeds (almonds, cashews, sunflower seeds, or hemp seeds) into a high-speed blender.
2. Add 1 cup water or coconut water.
3. OPTIONAL: Add 1 organic date (pre-soak 1 hour to soften) for sweetness and/or $1/3$ teaspoon vanilla extract for smoothness.
4. Blend on low to start and increase speed to high for 2-3 minutes, to finely pulverize the nuts or seeds and create a smooth texture.
5. OPTIONAL: Pour liquid through a cheesecloth-lined strainer or nut bag and hand squeeze the liquid through the cloth.
6. Use nut milk as a base for smoothies, a liquid in whole grains, or a tasty beverage.

6 Nut and Seed Milk Tips

1. **3:1 Ratio.** Start with a ratio of 3 parts liquid to 1 part nuts or seeds. Use more or less liquid depending on your personal preference for smoothness.
2. **Make a Little at a Time.** Nut and seed milk stays fresh in the refrigerator for a few days.
3. **To Strain or Not to Strain. It's Up to You.** Strain the blended nut milk in cheesecloth, a nut bag, or a fine-mesh strainer. Straining ensures a smooth, milky texture, and you can use this nut or seed pulp as a base for other creations. Do not strain cashews, hemp seeds, and sesame seeds due to their soft texture. If you do not strain the nut or seed milk, the nutrients and fiber from the nuts or seeds go right into your smoothie.
4. **Pulp for Breakfast.** Add pulp from the nut milk to a whole grain breakfast.
5. **Dehydrate the Pulp.** Dehydrate the pulp to use in crackers or crusts, or grind it into gluten-free flour. To dehydrate, spread the pulp onto dehydrator sheets and dehydrate until crisp, about 4-6 hours. Blend in a food processor and sift to make flour.
6. **To Soak or Not to Soak. It's Up to You.** Many raw foodists pre-soak nuts and seeds to neutralize enzyme inhibitors, make proteins more readily available for absorption, and make digestion easier. From a culinary view, pre-soaked nuts and seeds are easier to blend and result in creamier milk. If you have not pre-soaked the nuts and seeds, you can still make quick nut milk, which works well with morning smoothies. Blend the milk, add fruit, re-blend, and you have a quick smoothie.

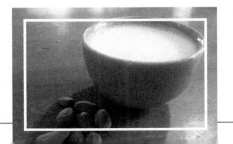

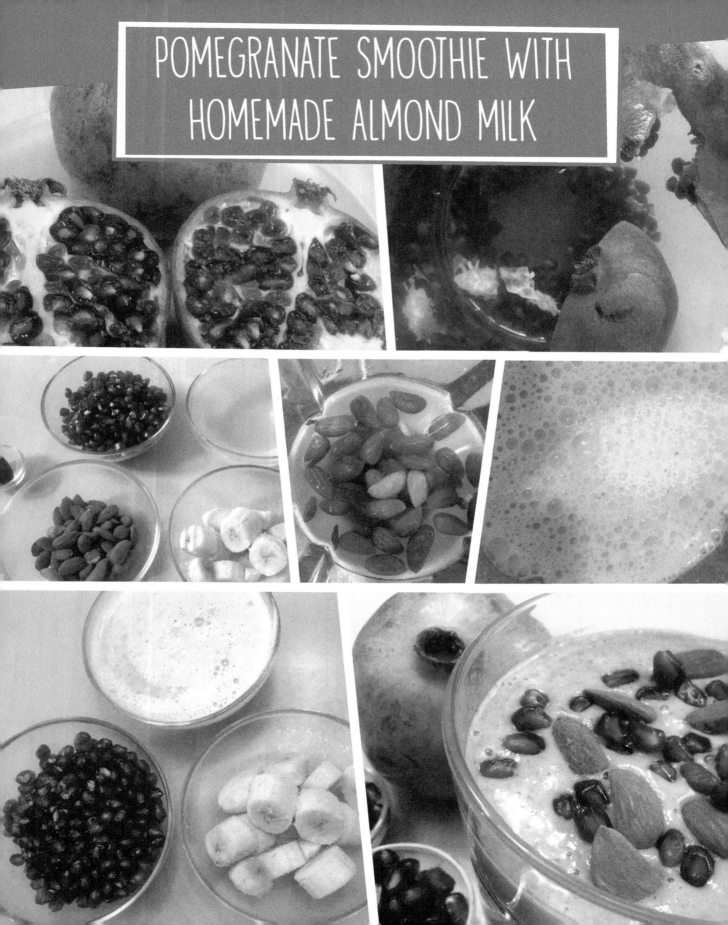

POMEGRANATE SMOOTHIE WITH HOMEMADE ALMOND MILK

Inspired by pomegranates sitting on my kitchen counter, I decided to create a smoothie. I wanted this smoothie to be special because I've loved sweet, juicy pomegranates since I was a young kid having fun mindfully picking the seeds out of the fruit like crabmeat, with the deep, red juice dripping down my arms.

Intuitively, I created the pomegranate smoothie with homemade almond milk, which is delicious even by itself. Enjoy the process of creating this thick, creamy, sweet smoothie.

SIMPLE INGREDIENTS

- 1 pomegranate, seeded
- 1 cup coconut water
- ½ cup almonds
- 1 Medjool date
- 1 frozen banana

SIMPLE STEPS

1. Simple Steps to Get the Seeds Out of a Pomegranate, Without All the Mess!
   - Cut pomegranate in half.
   - Place pomegranate in a bowl of cold water.
   - Tear apart the pomegranate with your hands. Seeds will float to the bottom of the bowl, and the tan membrane will rise to the top.
   - Mindfully examine the seeds and take out any small pieces of membrane.
2. Fresh Homemade Almond Milk
   - Blend coconut water, almonds, and date in a high-speed blender for 1-2 minutes.
   - Enjoy a taste.
3. My First-Ever Pomegranate Smoothie
   - Add banana to the almond milk in the blender and blend for about a minute.
   - Enjoy another taste.
   - Sprinkle in pomegranate seeds and blend for another minute.
   - Pour smoothie into a glass.
   - Top with a few pomegranate seeds and almonds to add crunch to the smoothie.
   - Enjoy! Enjoy! Enjoy!

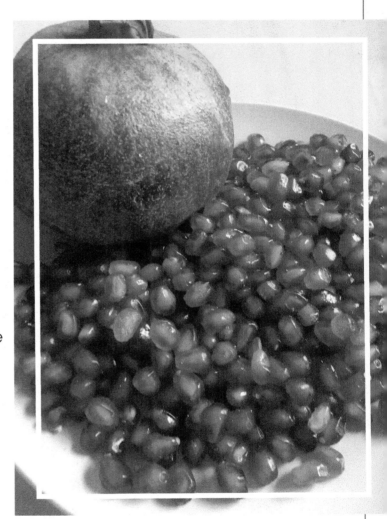

> " I previously thought nut milk was hard to make. Once learning how quick and easy it is to make nut milk, especially for my morning smoothies, I no longer buy store-bought milk. Since I'm such an advocate for eating and drinking real whole foods, this fits perfectly with my philosophy. "

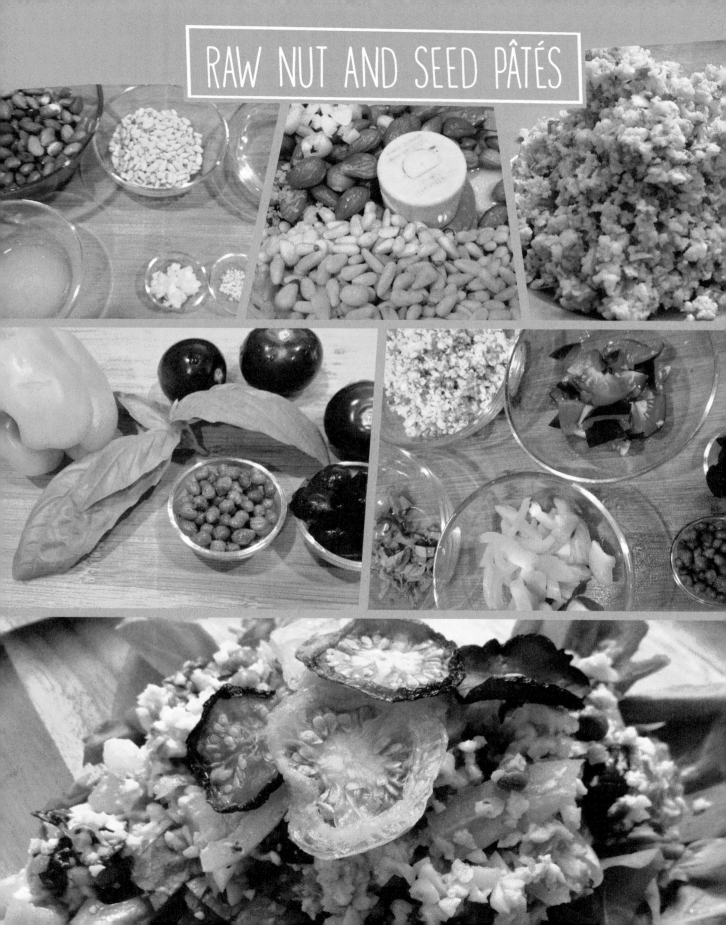

RAW NUT AND SEED PÂTÉS

Raw nut and seed pâtés are great base foundations for a variety of dishes. Enjoy pâtés as spreads or dips, on top of a salad, in a wrap, on veggies or crackers, or as a base for veggie burgers. Experiment by preparing a base nut and seed pâté, then intuitively add your own favorite fresh herbs and spices to create a variety of textures and flavors.

Similar to salad dressings, pâtés are made with a fat (nuts and/or seeds), an acid (citrus), and sea salt, then extras like fresh herbs and spices.

In this section, you'll learn how to make a basic almond pâté, a Mediterranean pâté with the almond base, a walnut pâté with fresh ginger, and an amazing raw taco.

Basic Almond Pâté

A rich almond pâté with pine nuts is a great base to experiment with different combinations of fresh herbs and spices.

SIMPLE INGREDIENTS

Pâté Base

- 1 ¼ cups raw almonds, soaked 2-3 hours in water, then drained
- ¾ cup raw pine nuts
- 2 cloves garlic
- 3 tbsp fresh lemon juice
- 1 tsp sea salt
- ½ cup water

Pâté Flavor Options

- 2 tbsp extra virgin olive oil
- ½ cup fresh basil
- ½ cup fresh sage
- 3 tbsp olives, pitted

SIMPLE STEPS

1. Gather mise en place.
2. To prepare the pâté base, pulse almonds, pine nuts, garlic, lemon juice, sea salt, and water in food processor until it reaches a coarse consistency.
3. Add your favorite flavors, such as olive oil, basil, sage, and/or olives, and blend.
4. Enjoy on crackers or veggies, in a wrap, or on top of a salad.

Mediterranean Almond Pâté with Heirloom Tomatoes, Kalamata Olives, Organic Capers

I love Kalamata olives and capers and intuitively created this Mediterranean pâté while studying with the Rouxbe Cooking School Plant-Based Professional Culinary Certification. This pâté was inspired by the beauty of the local Arizona orange sweet peppers, yellow and purple heirloom tomatoes, and home-garden basil, and accented with the saltiness of Kalamata olives and capers. I had so much fun intuitively creating this pâté. Hope you enjoy it.

1. **Make Raw Organic Almond and Pine Nut Pâté.** Blend in a food processor almonds (soaked for 3 hours), pine nuts, fresh garlic, lemon juice, sea salt, and a touch of organic extra virgin olive oil.

2. **Add Mediterranean accents.** Toss in orange peppers, heirloom tomatoes, fresh basil, capers, and Kalamata olives and capers.

3. **Mediterranean Almond Pâté Arugula Salad.** Enjoy the pâté on a bed of local Arizona arugula with dehydrated heirloom tomatoes.

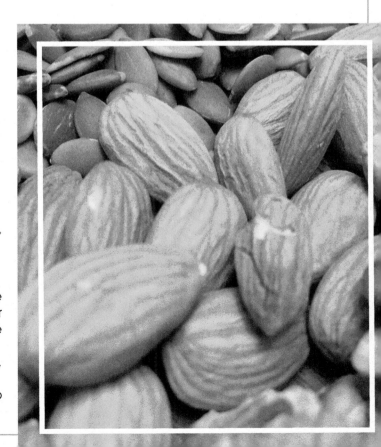

PECAN PÂTÉ WITH RED PEPPERS AND GINGER

Pecan pâté is another base foundation to create simple, unique pâtés with your favorite herbs and spices. You can also create this base pâté with walnuts.

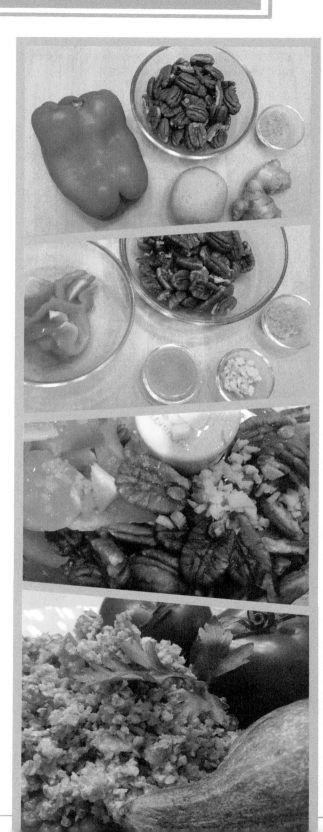

SIMPLE INGREDIENTS

- 2 cups pecans, soaked 2-3 hours, then drained
- ¼ cup fresh lemon juice
- ⅓ cup red bell pepper
- 1 inch fresh ginger root, minced
- 1 tsp sea salt

- Serving Extras
  - Lettuce or cabbage leaves
  - Tomatoes, onions, avocados
  - Flaxseed crackers
  - Fresh veggies
  - Tortilla wrap

SIMPLE STEPS

1. Gather your mise en place.
2. Place all ingredients in a food processor and blend until desired consistency is reached.
3. Serving Suggestions:
   - Serve in lettuce or cabbage leaf wraps, topped with tomatoes, onions, and avocados.
   - Use as a dip with flaxseed crackers or veggies.
   - Enjoy in a tortilla wrap.

5 Tips to Shop for and Enjoy Nuts and Seeds

1. **Raw.** Eat raw, whole, unsalted nuts and seeds. They are whole foods and not processed.

2. **No added oils.** Be sure to read labels and buy nuts, seeds, and nut butters with no added pro-inflammatory omega-6-rich oils like cottonseed, peanut, safflower, and sunflower.

3. **Keep cold.** Store in the refrigerator, as nuts and seeds may go rancid due to their high fat content.

4. **Eat fresh nuts and seeds.** Do not eat nuts or seeds that smell and taste bad (like oil paint); they may be carcinogenic.

5. **Be careful.** Toasted, chopped, and ground nuts go rancid more quickly than whole raw nuts, so eat them as soon as they are prepped.

Raw Taco Salad

This raw taco salad is a pâté with favorite taco seasonings. Enjoy the raw taco wrapped in a red cabbage leaf for a delicious lunch or picnic.

SIMPLE INGREDIENTS

Nut Taco Filling

- 2 cups almonds, soaked 4 hours in water
- 2 cups walnuts, soaked 4 hours in water
- 1 tsp sea salt
- 1 fresh lime, zest and juice
- ¼ cup fresh cilantro, chopped
- ¼ cup yellow onion, finely diced
- 1 tbsp garlic, minced
- ½ cup taco seasoning (recipe)

Taco Seasoning

- 2 tbsp coriander seeds, freshly ground
- 2 tbsp cumin seeds, freshly ground
- 2 tbsp paprika
- 2 tbsp chili powder
- 2 tbsp dried oregano
- 1 tbsp ancho seasoning
- 1 tbsp black pepper
- ½ tbsp sea salt

SIMPLE STEPS

1. Gather mise en place.
2. Pre-soak almonds and walnuts.
3. Soak almonds and walnuts separately with ½ tsp sea salt and ½ gallon water.
4. After soaking, drain and rinse well.
5. Spread nuts on a parchment-paper-lined sheet pan and dry overnight.
6. Prepare taco seasoning.
7. Combine all ingredients in a bowl and mix well.
8. Mix taco filling.
9. Place almonds and walnuts into food processor and pulse until nuts are small (about ⅛-inch) pieces.
10. Pour the almonds and nuts into a large bowl.
11. Add all of the other ingredients, including the taco seasoning, and toss well.
12. Enjoy wrapped in a red cabbage leaf.

Quick and Easy Steps to Make Nut Butter

Simple Almond Butter

Once you make your own almond butter at home, you'll want to make it all the time. It's easy, less expensive than store-bought jars, and tastes great. It's so mindful to see almonds transform into almond butter.

1. Pour about a cup of raw organic almonds into a high-speed blender or food processor.
2. Turn on blender, moving from low to high.
3. Check almonds every 4-5 minutes for consistency.
4. Push the almonds down into the blade as needed.
5. Blend until smooth and you will see the oil from the almonds.
6. Enjoy with a fresh organic apple.

Top 5 Ways to Enjoy Seeds Every Day

1. **Buy fresh seeds.** Shop in the bulk section of your grocery store and store seeds in your refrigerator so that they stay fresh and do not go rancid.

2. **Grind flaxseeds.** Hand-grind flaxseeds to enhance the absorption of the seeds' nutrients in your body.

3. **Add to smoothies**. Add chia seeds, hemp seeds, or ground flaxseeds to your breakfast smoothies. Try almond milk or hemp milk, frozen bananas, raspberries, and blueberries and sprinkle seeds into the smoothie.

4. **Enjoy with veggies.** Sprinkle seeds on raw salads, veggie stir-fries, and roasted vegetables to add crunch, flavor, and texture.

5. **Whole grains.** Add seeds to your morning grains. Try steel-cut oats with all kinds of nuts (almonds, walnuts, cashews) and some seeds (chia, hemp, and/or flaxseeds).

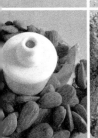
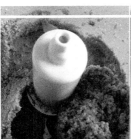
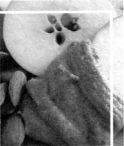

HEMP SEED TABOULI

Refreshing, light tabouli featuring protein-rich hemp seeds is a perfect alternative to traditional tabouli made with gluten grain bulgur. Enjoy the natural aroma of the fresh parsley, mint, and lemon juice. After you have learned the simple foundation recipe to make gluten-free tabouli, have fun experimenting with different fresh herbs, such as lemon basil, and different varieties of beautiful heirloom tomatoes.

SIMPLE INGREDIENTS

- 2 bunches fresh parsley
- ¼ cup fresh mint
- ½ cup hemp seeds
- 1 large tomato, diced
- ¼ cup fresh lemon juice
- 2 tbsp organic extra virgin olive oil
- 2 tbsp onions, chopped
- 1 tsp sea salt

SIMPLE STEPS

1. Place parsley and mint in a food processor and pulse several times until well chopped.
2. Transfer to a mixing bowl and add the hemp seeds, tomato, lemon juice, olive oil, onion, and salt.
3. Toss and serve.
4. Enjoy!

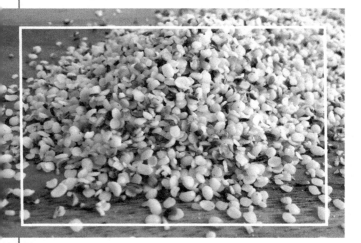

Get Clear on Plant-Based Omega-3

Omega-3s for Health

- Essential fatty acids (EFAs) are necessary for optimal health; they are essential for the structure and function of cells, brain function, metabolism, the immune system, and the nervous system.
- Our bodies cannot make them, so we must eat them.
- ALA, alpha-linolenic acid, the omega-3 in seeds, is partially converted into DHA and EPA in the body.

Omega-3-Rich Seeds

Some seeds are high in omega-3 fatty acids, which reduce inflammation, boost brain and cardiovascular health, and decrease the risk of type 2 diabetes.

Seeds High in Omega-3 Fatty Acids (grams in 1 ounce)

Flaxseeds	6.3
Chia seeds	4.9
Hemp seeds	2.8 (high in protein, 10.3 grams/ounce)

Why Eat Hemp Seeds (Hemp Hearts)

- Great vegetarian protein
- Complete protein, contains all nine essential amino acids
- Boost immune system and hasten recovery
- Natural anti-inflammatory
- Repair soft tissue damage and speed recovery caused by physical activity
- Enhance fat metabolism
- Easy to digest

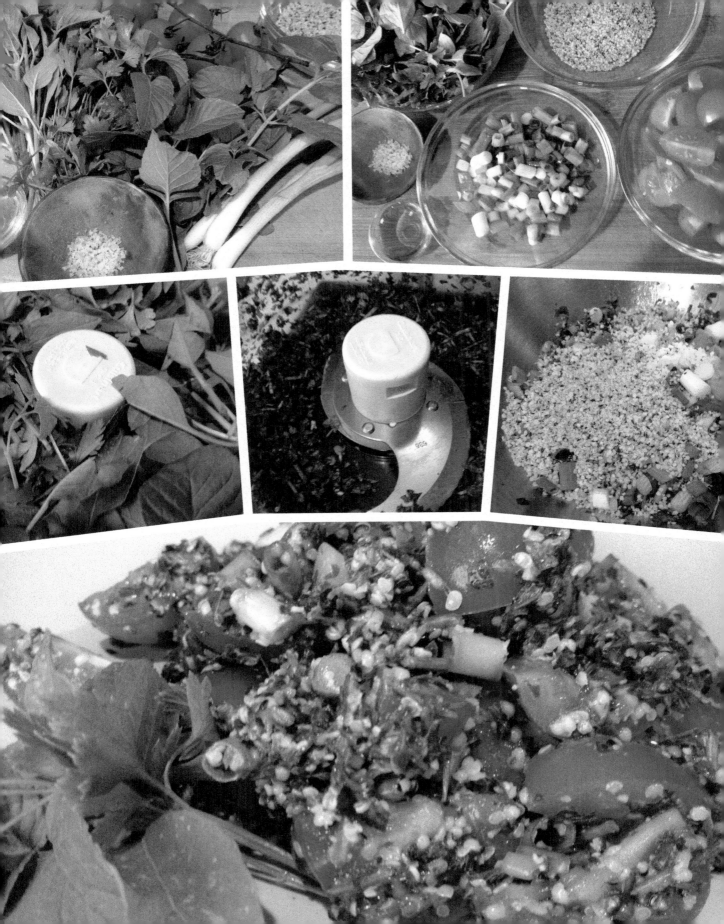

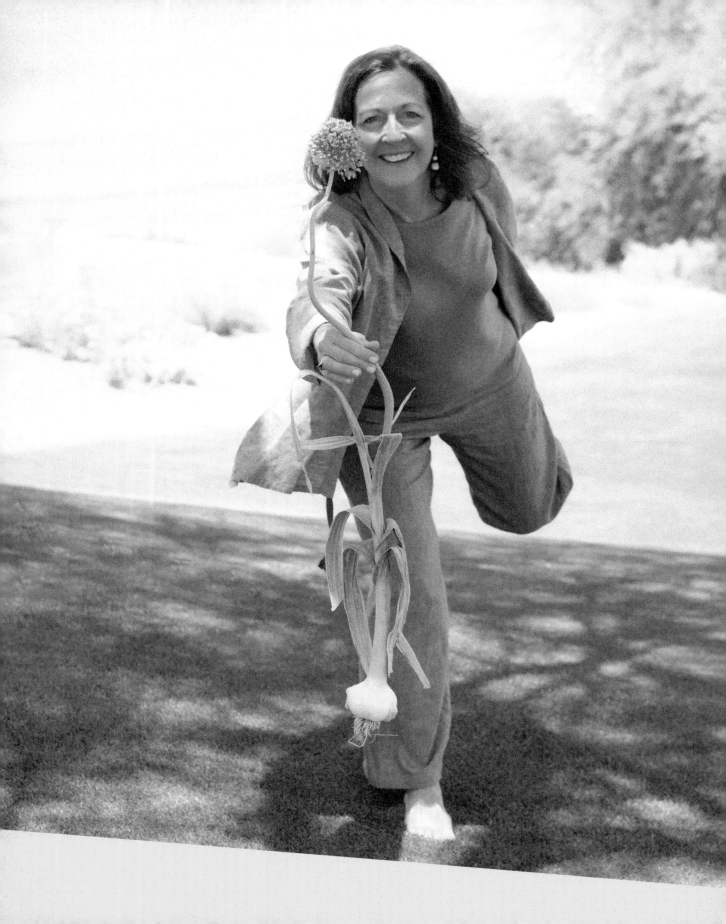

Dehydrated Raw Flaxseed Crackers

Flax seeds, chia seeds, and buckwheat groats are perfect for a flatbread batter because they form a natural mucilaginous gel when combined with water. Once dried, it's a great binder for crackers, flatbread, and raw tortillas or wraps.

5 Ingredients for Dehydrated Flatbread

The basic ingredients to create the base for dehydrated flatbread or crisp crackers are very simple. Have fun using your intuition to create your own versions of crackers with this raw dehydrating process.

1. Soaked flax seeds, chia seeds, or buckwheat groats
2. Fresh vegetables (peppers, tomatoes, beets, carrots) or fruit (apples, pears)
3. Nuts or seeds (almonds, cashews, pecans, sunflower seeds)
4. Herbs and spices (basil, oregano, ginger, turmeric)
5. Dehydrator: to dry for 8-12 hours

Sweet Pepper Almond Flax Crisp

SIMPLE INGREDIENTS

- ½ cup golden flax seeds, ground, then soaked in 1 ½ cups water for ½ hour
- ¾ cup raw almonds, soaked in water for 2-3 hours, drained
- 1 ¼ cup yellow bell pepper, minced
- 1 shallot, minced
- ½ cup sun-dried tomatoes, soaked and drained
- 1 ½ tsp chili powder
- 1 ½ tsp onion granules
- 1 tsp sea salt

SIMPLE STEPS

1. Gather mise en place.
2. Blend ingredients.
   - Add soaked flax meal (ground flaxseeds and water) and almonds to food processor and blend until smooth.
   - Remove and place in mixing bowl.
   - Blend yellow pepper, shallot, and sun-dried tomatoes with a touch of water.
   - Add chili powder, onion granules, and sea salt to food processor with the pepper, shallot, and sun-dried tomatoes until smooth.
   - Add vegetable mixture to the bowl with flax meal and almonds and fold together until thoroughly combined.

3. Dehydrate.
   - Set dehydrator at 115 degrees F.
   - Spoon mixture onto dehydrator tray. Spread mixture evenly to ¼-inch thickness on non-stick dehydrator sheets with an off-set spatula.
   - Dehydrate 1-2 hours. Once partially dried, score batter to desired size and shape.
   - Dehydrate an additional 1-3 hours. Flip the crackers so they dry properly.
   - Dehydrate an additional 1-2 hours or until crackers are crisp.
   - Dehydrating time depends on how thick the paste is to begin and how crisp you want the crackers.

4. Options.
   - Soft taco shells: Once flipped onto the dehydrator screen, dehydrate for 1-2 hours or until batter is not wet and is pliable.
   - If crisps dry too much, sprinkle water to restore pliability.
   - Enjoy as a cracker snack, dip in hummus, or top with a pâté.

Action : Experiment with Nuts and Seeds

In this section, we've explored several ways to enjoy nuts and seeds: making your own milk and nut butter, creating pâtés with various herbs and spices for spreads, snacks, and salads, preparing gluten-free hemp seed tabouli, and dehydrating raw flaxseed crackers. I invite you to have fun intuitively experimenting with one or two culinary methods of using nuts and seeds in beverages and beautiful tasty dishes.

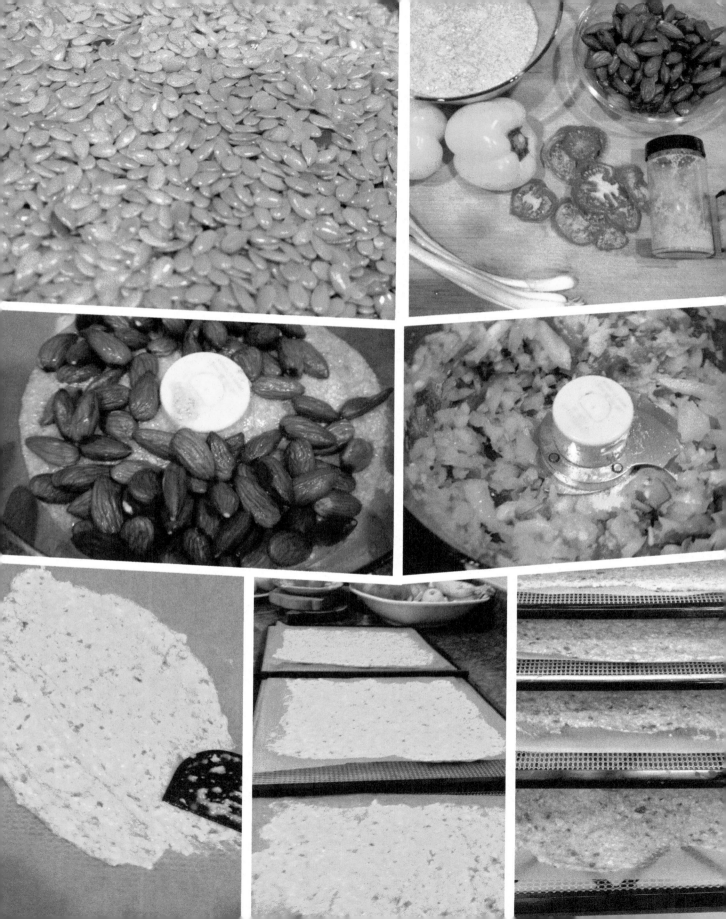

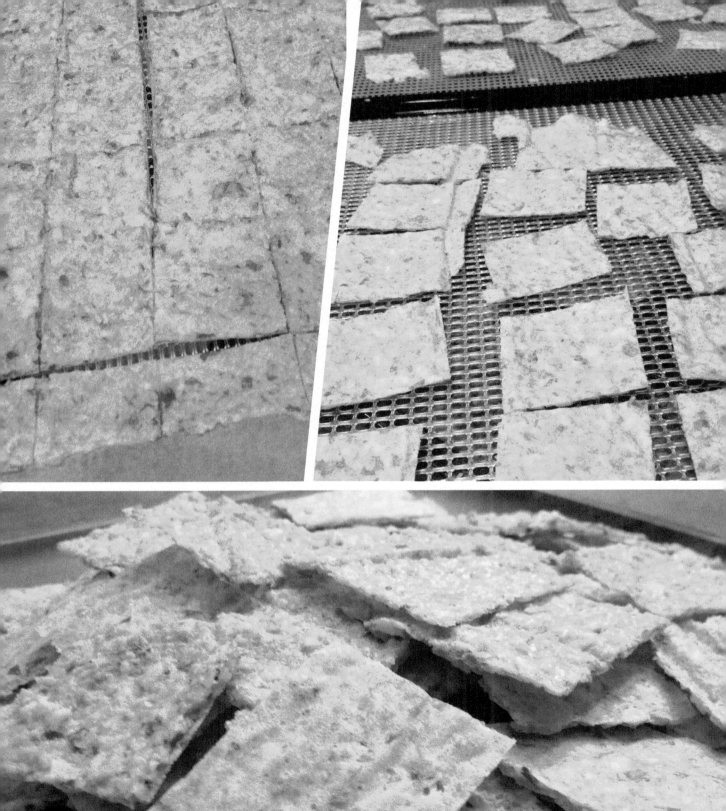

Create Healthy Gourmet Desserts and Snacks and Enjoy Superfoods

Culinary
- 5 superfood snacks always in my pantry
- 4 ways to enjoy chocolate
- 5 tips to make your own unique delicious sorbet
- Simple steps to create fruit sorbet
- 6 favorite natural sweeteners
- 5 ways to enjoy organic sprouted spelt flatbread

Recipes
- Chocolate Avocado Pudding
- Vegan Chocolate Cream Pie
- Chocolate Sweet Potato Brownie
- Raw Chocolate Bliss
- Raspberry Cara Cara Orange Sorbet
- Raw Carrot Cake
- Rosemary Citrus Olives
- Organic Sprouted Spelt Flatbread

Nutrition
- Get clear on superfoods
- Benefits of dark chocolate
- Get to know goji berries
- 6 reasons why you can eat dark chocolate

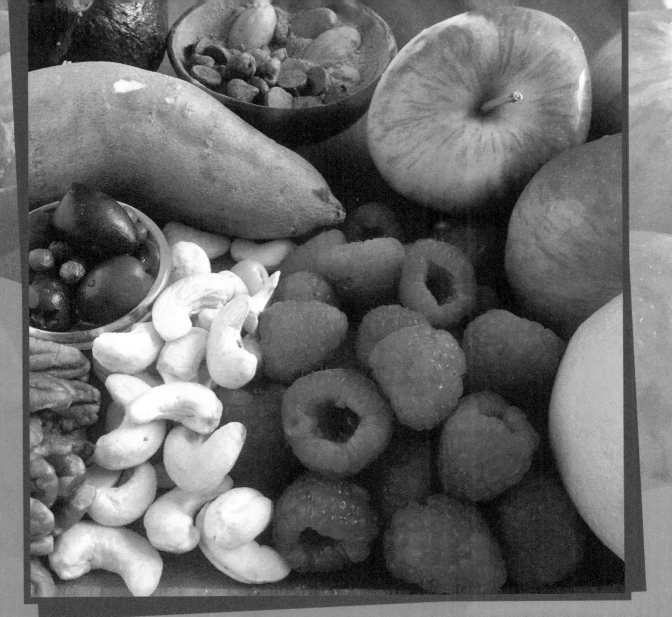

CREATE HEALTHY GOURMET DESSERTS AND SNACKS AND ENJOY SUPERFOODS

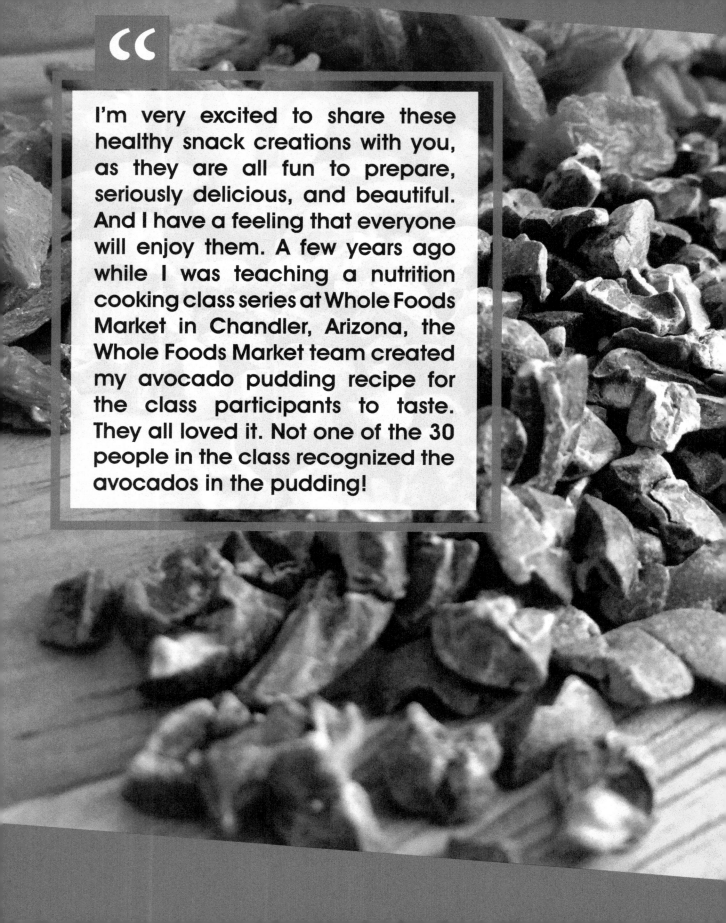

"

I'm very excited to share these healthy snack creations with you, as they are all fun to prepare, seriously delicious, and beautiful. And I have a feeling that everyone will enjoy them. A few years ago while I was teaching a nutrition cooking class series at Whole Foods Market in Chandler, Arizona, the Whole Foods Market team created my avocado pudding recipe for the class participants to taste. They all loved it. Not one of the 30 people in the class recognized the avocados in the pudding!

DESSERTS AND SNACKS ARE ALWAYS EXCITING

Really enjoy dessert

It's fun to create and enjoy eating beautiful, delicious, healthy desserts, snacks, and superfoods. We'll explore chocolate, superfoods, and raw and cooked desserts with unique ingredients, such as a brownie made with a sweet potato. We'll also create savory snacks with olives, kale, and an easy sprouted spelt flatbread.

We will explore:
- The benefits of dark chocolate
- Superfood snacks

You'll learn how to:
- Create incredible chocolate desserts
  - Rich, creamy chocolate avocado pudding
  - Vegan chocolate cream pie with tofu
  - Chocolate sweet potato brownie
  - Raw chocolate bliss with raw cacao powder
- Make refreshing fruit sorbet with in-season fresh fruit
- Create a tasty, beautiful raw carrot cake
- Prepare mouth-watering savory snacks
  - Olives with rosemary infusion
  - Organic sprouted spelt flatbread

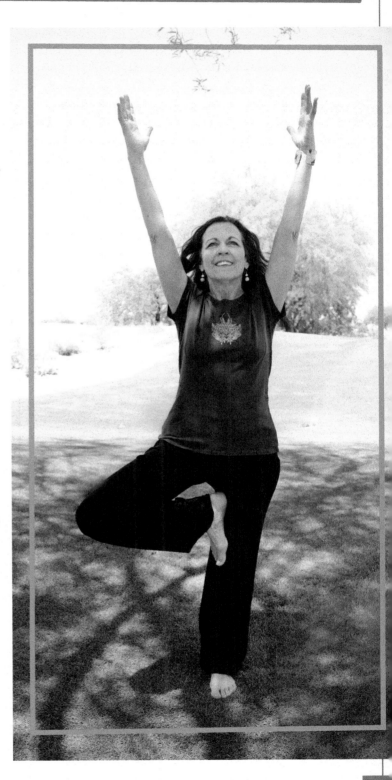

GET CLEAR ON SUPERFOOD SNACKS

According to the Oxford Dictionary, a superfood is "a nutrient-rich food considered to be especially beneficial for health and well-being."

Superfoods are trendy, but many superfoods have been around for centuries. I was introduced to superfoods in 2006 by David Wolfe, who is a leading international raw food expert and one of my favorite instructors at the Institute for Integrative Nutrition (IIN). According to Wolfe, superfoods are vibrant, nutritionally dense foods that have recently become widely available and that offer tremendous dietary and healing potential.

I still clearly remember the day when Wolfe was lecturing about superfoods and mentioned raw cacao and goji berries as great snacks. During our lunch break, my IIN friends and I literally ran to Whole Foods Market to buy cacao nibs and goji berries, and I've been eating them ever since. Today, they are both a staple in my kitchen for desserts and morning smoothies.

Get to Know Goji Berries (Wolfberries)

- Used in traditional Chinese medicine for thousands of years
- Traditionally known as a strength-building, longevity, and immune system superfood
- Grown in South America and the Himalayas
- High in protein, with 18 amino acids, including all eight essential amino acids
- Rich in antioxidants and more than 20 trace minerals, and full of fiber

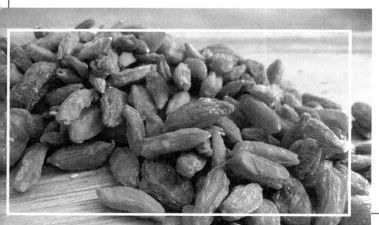

5 Superfood Snacks Always in My Pantry

1. **Goji berries (wolfberries).** Antioxidant and protein-rich, with a strong, sweet, bitter taste. Enjoy a handful as a crunchy snack. Blend in smoothies or add as a topping. Cook in a veggie stir-fry. Enjoy as a sweet, earthy, warm tea.

2. **Raw cacao.** Full of antioxidants, potassium, and magnesium. Enjoy 2 ounces of dark chocolate every day. Buy a bar with 70% cacao. If that's too bitter for you, start with 55% cacao and enjoy.

3. **Ginger.** Ginger chews, made from ginger root, are the perfect chewy snack with benefits. Tasty bits of ginger with natural anti-inflammatory powers. Ginger may reduce nausea and joint pain, aid in the recovery of soft-tissue injuries, and help promote faster healing of strains.

4. **Chia seeds.** Rich source of plant-based omega-3 fatty acids, full of protein, antioxidants, and minerals. Chia seeds contain soluble and insoluble fiber and expand to 12 times their size. Enjoy chia seeds in smoothies or raw puddings, or with cooked whole grains. For an egg substitute in baking, use 1 teaspoon of chia seeds and 3 teaspoons of water for 1 egg.

5. **Hemp seeds (hemp hearts).** A complete protein, contains all nine essential amino acids, which boost the immune system and hasten recovery. Rich in omega-3 and omega-6 fatty acids. According to vegan triathlete Brandan Brazier, in his book "Thrive Foods," hemp seeds have natural anti-inflammatory properties, key factors for speeding the repair of soft tissue damage caused by physical activity. Brazier also writes that top-quality protein, such as hemp, is instrumental in muscle tissue regeneration and fat metabolism, enhances fat metabolism, and is easy to digest. Enjoy hemp seeds as a snack, make hemp seed milk, or sprinkle on a smoothie, whole grain breakfast, salad or roasted veggies.

6 Reasons Why You Can Eat Dark Chocolate

1. Good for Heart Health

- Studies show that eating a small amount of dark chocolate two or three times every week can help lower blood pressure.
- Dark chocolate improves blood flow and may help prevent the formation of blood clots.
- Eating dark chocolate may prevent arteriosclerosis (hardening of the arteries).

2. Good for the Brain

- Because dark chocolate increases blood flow to the brain, it may contribute to improved cognitive function. Dark chocolate may also help reduce the risk of stroke.
- Dark chocolate contains several chemical compounds that may positively affect mood and cognitive health. Because chocolate contains phenylethylamine (PEA), which encourages the brain to release endorphins, it may make us feel happier.
- Dark chocolate contains caffeine, a mild stimulant. However, dark chocolate contains much less caffeine than coffee does. A 1.5-ounce bar of dark chocolate contains 27 mg of caffeine, compared to 200 mg in eight ounces of coffee.

3. Helps Control Blood Sugar

- Dark chocolate helps keep blood vessels healthy and improves circulation to protect against Type 2 diabetes.
- Flavonoids in dark chocolate help reduce insulin resistance by helping cells function normally and regain the ability to use insulin efficiently.
- Dark chocolate has a low glycemic index and glycemic load, meaning that it won't cause huge spikes in blood sugar levels.

4. Full of Antioxidants

- Antioxidants cleanse the body of free radicals, which cause oxidative damage to the cells. Free radicals are also associated with the aging process and may be a cause of cancer; thus, eating antioxidant-rich foods like dark chocolate may be cancer protective and slow the signs of aging.

5. Contains Theobromine

- Theobromine has been shown to harden tooth enamel. That means that dark chocolate, unlike most other sweets, lowers your risk of getting cavities if you practice proper dental hygiene.

6. High in Vitamins and Minerals

- The copper and potassium in dark chocolate help prevent stroke and cardiovascular ailments.
- The iron in chocolate protects against iron deficiency anemia.
- The magnesium in chocolate helps prevent Type 2 diabetes, high blood pressure, and heart disease.

4 Ways to Enjoy Chocolate

Dark chocolate is distinguished by the percentage of cacao solids in the bar. The higher the percentage of cacao in a chocolate bar, the lower the amount of sugar.

1. **Dark Chocolate Bar:** Made with 70% cacao. If you are new to the bitter taste of dark chocolate, start with a 55% cacao chocolate bar. As you become accustomed to the flavor, try chocolate with higher levels of cacao.
2. **Raw Chocolate:** Raw cacao is extracted from fermented cacao beans, which are dried without roasting or roasted at low temperatures.
3. **Cacao Nibs:** Cacao bean crushed into little pieces. Try a few cacao nibs and experience their bitterness. Add nibs to smoothies or chocolate desserts.
4. **Cacao Bean:** The actual bean or seed. It's definitely an acquired taste; try a bite.

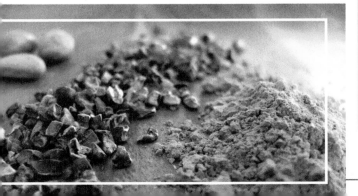

DELICIOUS GUILT-FREE CHOCOLATE RECIPES

Enjoy creating vegan, gluten-free chocolate recipes with fruit, raw cacao powder, nuts, natural sweeteners, and even sweet potatoes. If you are a chocolate lover or have a sweet tooth, try these "good-for-us" chocolate desserts.

Vegan Chocolate Cream Pie

Try this simple chocolate dessert recipe that everyone enjoys. This gourmet-quality pie is so much fun to make and is beautiful and delicious every time I teach it in my private and group cooking classes. Learn to quickly and easily melt chocolate chips right in your oven. If you have extra chocolate pie, cut it into small pieces and freeze for snacks.

SIMPLE INGREDIENTS

Crust
- 2 cups raw pecans
- ¼ cup maple sugar
- 1 ½ tbsp coconut oil
- ½ tsp sea salt

Filling
- 2 ½ cups vegan dark chocolate chips
- 2 packages organic soft silken tofu (260g packages)
- 1 tsp vanilla extract or 1 vanilla bean, scraped
- Pinch of sea salt

SIMPLE STEPS

1. Make the Crust.
   - Pulse pecans and maple sugar in food processor.
   - Add coconut oil and sea salt.
   - Pulse to combine well.
   - Press and shape mixture into the bottom of a 10-inch springform pan.
2. Melt Chocolate Chips.
   - Preheat oven to 350 degrees F.
   - Pour the chocolate chips in a single layer onto a flat baking sheet.
   - Place in the oven to melt for no more than 3-4 minutes or until melted. Be careful that you don't burn them.
3. Blend the Filling.
   - Place tofu, vanilla, sea salt, and melted chocolate chips into a food processor.
   - Blend until smooth.
   - Pour mixture into pie crust and chill for at least 30 minutes.
   - Top with fresh fruit and nuts.
   - Enjoy.

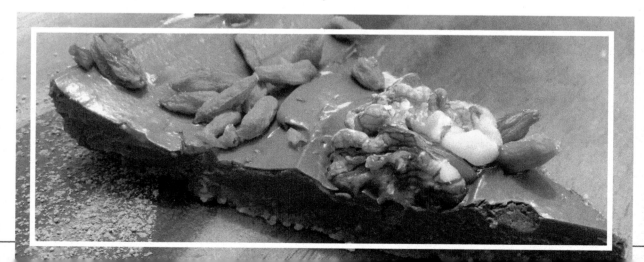

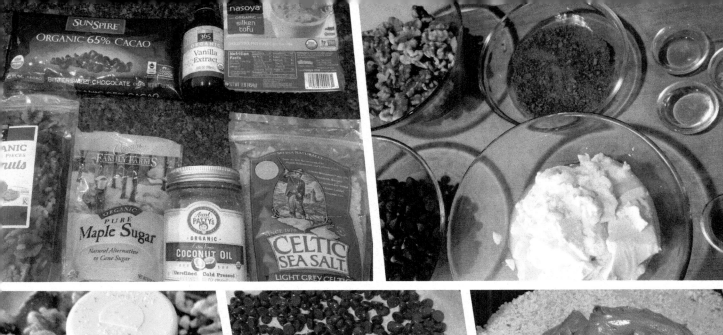

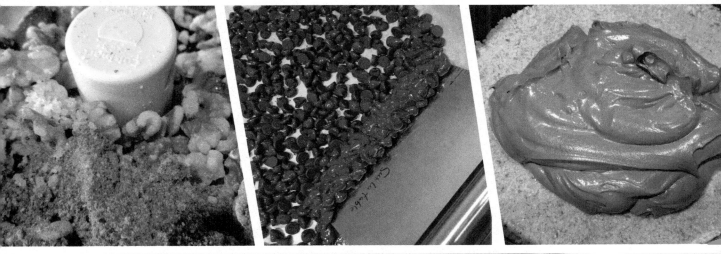

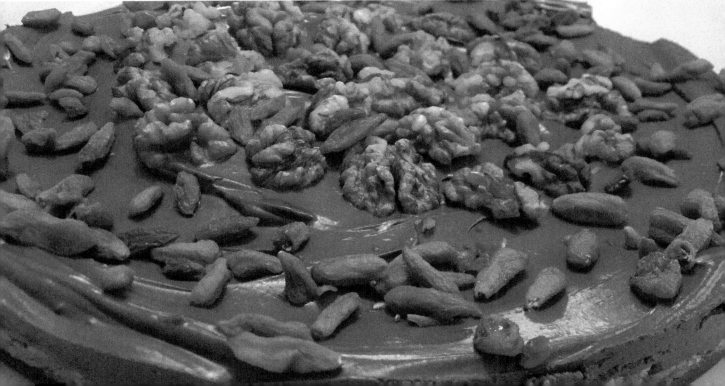

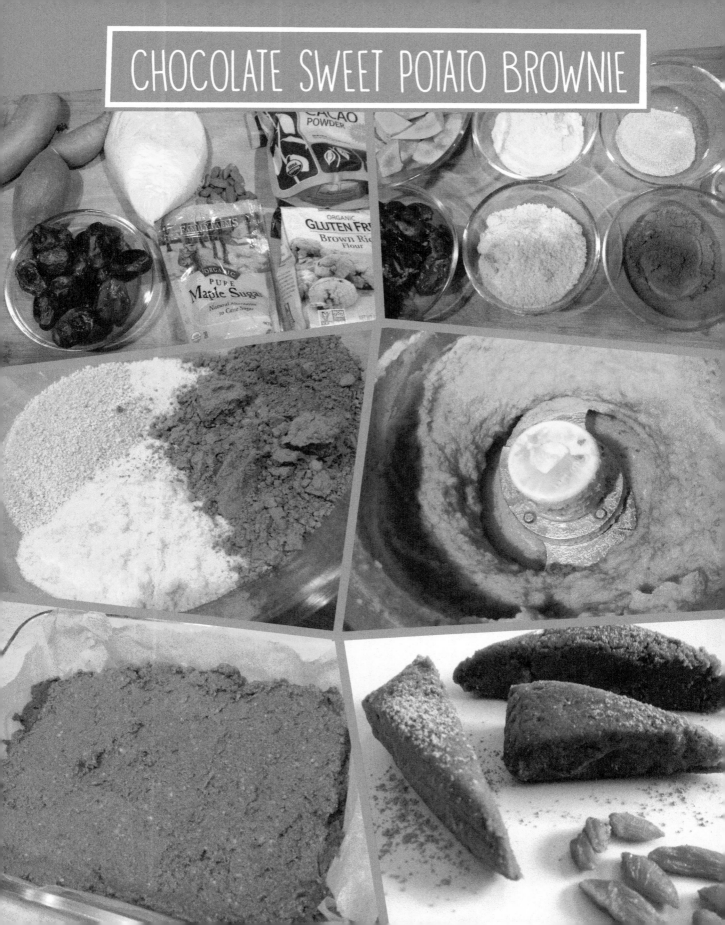

CHOCOLATE SWEET POTATO BROWNIE

Delicious vegan, gluten-free chocolate dessert made with a sweet root veggie, the sweet potato. This brownie is always a favorite at kids' and adults' cooking classes. It's one of those desserts we can even eat for breakfast!

SIMPLE INGREDIENTS

- 2 medium to large sweet potatoes
- 12 Medjool dates, pitted
- ²⁄₃ cup raw almonds, ground
- ½ cup brown rice flour
- 4 tbsp raw cacao
- 3 tbsp maple sugar
- Pinch sea salt

SIMPLE STEPS

1. Pre-heat oven to 350 F.
2. Peel sweet potatoes, cut into chunks, and steam in a bamboo steamer for about 20 minutes until they become really soft.
3. Once sweet potatoes are soft and beginning to fall apart, remove from steamer.
4. Mix sweet potatoes and pitted dates into food processor and blend.
5. Put remaining ingredients into a large bowl and stir to combine.
6. Add sweet potato/date mixture to other ingredients and stir well.
7. Place mixture into 8-inch by 8-inch parchment-paper-lined baking dish.
8. Cook for about 20 minutes.
9. Test doneness by pushing a toothpick into the brownie. The brownie is ready when a toothpick comes out dry.
10. Allow baking dish to cool for about 10 minutes.
11. Remove the brownies from baking dish.
12. Cool for a few minutes and cut into pieces.
13. Enjoy!

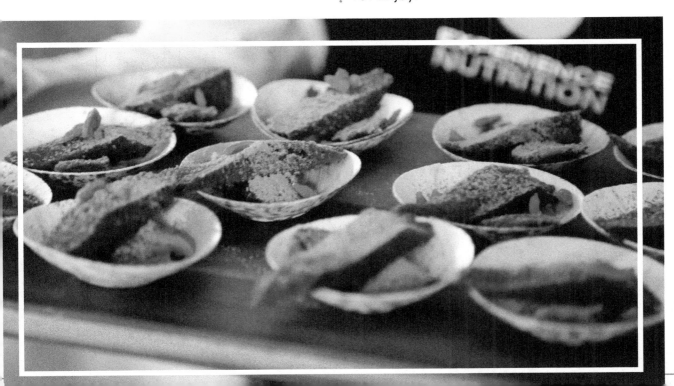

CHOCOLATE AVOCADO PUDDING

Incredible, rich, and creamy vegan chocolate pudding will delight everyone. Make it for dessert or an after-work or after-school snack. Once you've made this avocado pudding, experiment by adding some extras, such as bananas, raspberries, blueberries, strawberries, homemade nut milk, and freshly ground spices, like cinnamon and nutmeg.

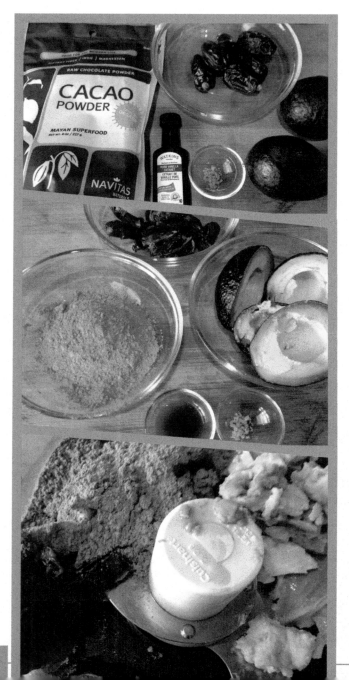

SIMPLE INGREDIENTS

- 4 ripe avocados
- 8 Medjool dates, pitted and sliced
- 2 tsp vanilla extract or 2 vanilla beans, scraped
- ½ cup raw cacao powder
- 2 cups water

SIMPLE STEPS

1. Place all ingredients in high-speed blender.
2. Blend on high for about 2 minutes.
3. Stop and scrape down sides of blender, if needed.
4. Blend for another 2 minutes or until completely pureed and smooth.
5. Refrigerate for 1-2 hours.
6. Enjoy topped with fresh fruit, nuts, and seeds.

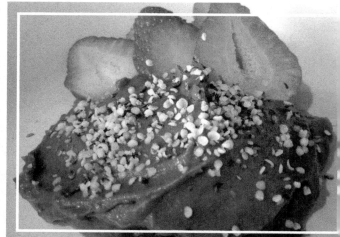

Raw Chocolate Bliss

Enjoy this rich, intense raw chocolate dessert, created with raw cacao powder, local Arizona dates, fresh raw almond butter, and vanilla bean, on a pecan maple sugar cinnamon crust.

Raw Pecan Cinnamon Crust

SIMPLE INGREDIENTS

- 1 ½ cups raw pecans
- 3 tbsp maple sugar
- ½ tsp sea salt
- ½ tbsp cinnamon, freshly ground

SIMPLE STEPS

1. Blend all ingredients in food processor until finely minced.
2. Press crust into 10-inch springform pan using your palms.

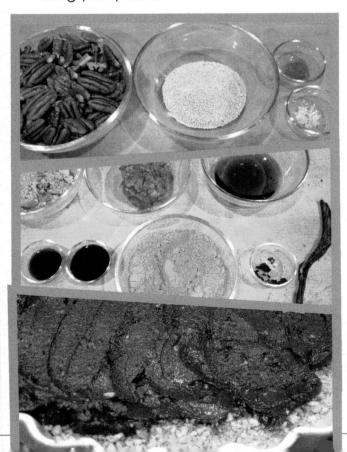

Chocolate Filling

SIMPLE INGREDIENTS

- ½ cup raw almond butter
- ½ cup date paste
- ¼ cup agave nectar or maple syrup
- 1 ½ tbsp tamari (gluten-free soy sauce)
- 1 cup raw cacao powder
- 1 vanilla bean, scraped
- ½ to 1 cup water

SIMPLE STEPS

1. Gather mise en place.
2. Make almond butter. Place raw almonds in food processor and blend until smooth and creamy.
3. Blend date paste. Soak dates in water for 1-2 hours until soft and pliable. Pour off water. Add to high-speed blender and top with water to cover fruit. Blend starting on low, then moving to high, until smooth.
4. Blend all ingredients in food processor until smooth and thick.
5. Add water if difficult to blend.
6. Pour filling into crust.
7. To set, freeze for about 20 minutes or refrigerate for an hour.
8. Slice. Use a knife dipped in hot water for a few seconds, wipe water away, then slice.
9. Plate with fruit or sorbet.
10. Enjoy.

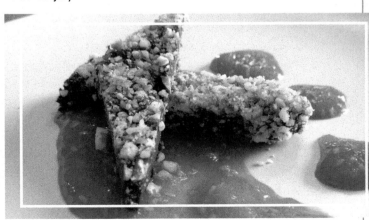

FRUIT SORBET

For most of my life I ate refreshing sorbet only at restaurants. Now with this simple sorbet process, I enjoy making it at home with local, seasonal fruit. I especially love sorbet with freshly harvested Arizona oranges. Intuitively create sorbet with fruits that are local and in season and experiment with different fruit, spices, and herbs to create sorbet year-round.

Simple Steps to Create Fruit Sorbet

SIMPLE INGREDIENTS

- 4 cups fresh fruit
- ½ cup fresh fruit juice, as needed
- Freshly ground spices or herbs
- Pinch sea salt
- 5 tbsp agave nectar or coconut sugar, as needed

SIMPLE STEPS

1. Blend fresh fruit, fresh fruit juice, ground spices or herbs, and a pinch of sea salt in high-speed blender.
2. Taste and add sweetener if needed.
3. Pour into frozen sorbet maker and process for about 15-20 minutes until thick, soft, and creamy.
4. For firmer sorbet, freeze in an air-tight container for about 2 hours and remove from freezer 15 minutes before serving.
5. Enjoy.

Raspberry Cara Cara Orange Sorbet

Sweet, refreshing sorbet features organic raspberries, local Arizona Cara Cara navel oranges, and a touch of nutmeg. Cara Cara oranges are one of my favorites, with their rosy interior and sweet taste. Pair this refreshing sorbet with shaved organic dark chocolate.

SIMPLE INGREDIENTS

- 4 cups fresh organic raspberries
- 5 tbsp agave nectar
- ½ Cara Cara navel orange, juiced
- Pinch sea salt
- Pinch freshly ground nutmeg
- 70% organic dark chocolate bar, shaved

SIMPLE STEPS

1. Blend all ingredients in high-speed blender.
2. Pour into frozen sorbet maker and process for about 15-20 minutes until thickened, soft, and creamy.
3. Sprinkle shaved dark chocolate on sorbet.
4. Serve and enjoy.

5 Tips to Make Your Own Unique, Delicious Sorbet

1. **Peak sweetness.** Use high-quality, fresh organic fruits at their peak of sweetness. The freezing process in making sorbet reduces the sweetness of fruit.
2. **Experiment.** Have fun making sorbet with all types of in-season fruit. Berries (blackberries, blueberries, raspberries, strawberries), stone fruit (cherries, peaches, plums), bananas, grapes, pears, oranges, and pineapple.
3. **Natural sweetener.** If the fruit tastes tart, add a sweetener such as agave nectar or coconut sugar.
4. **Citrus.** Add a squeeze of citrus to balance flavor or add acidity.
5. **Accent.** Experiment with spices such as freshly ground cinnamon or nutmeg, fresh herbs such as basil or mint, citrus zest, or vanilla.

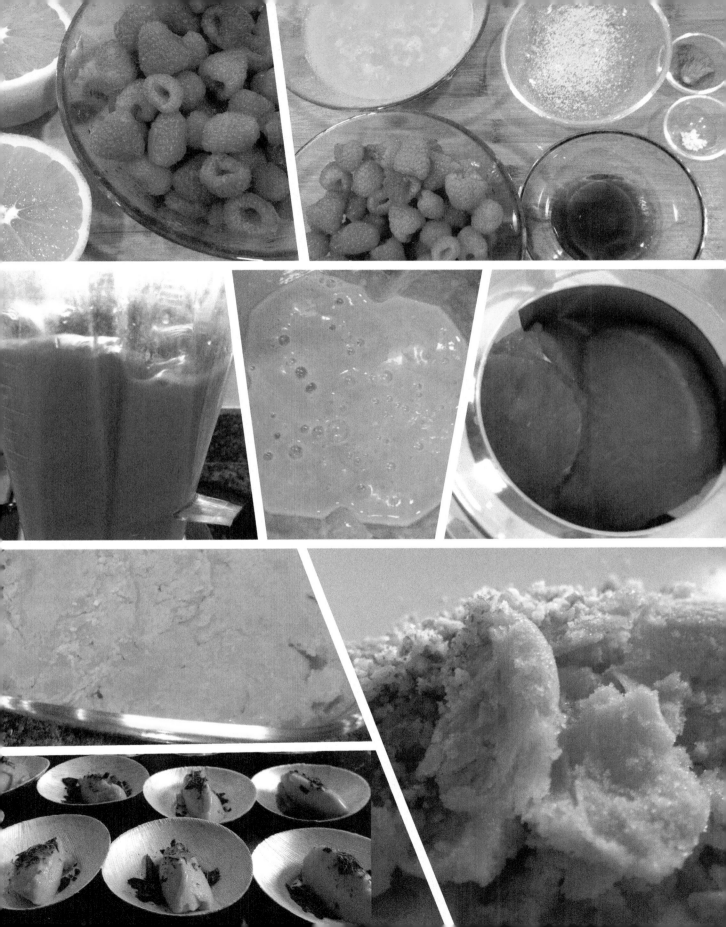

RAW CARROT CAKE

Carrot cake has been a favorite of mine for decades. As much as I love the aromatherapy of cooking raisins with cinnamon and nutmeg for a baked carrot cake, I love the simplicity and freshness of a raw version of carrot cake.

SIMPLE INGREDIENTS

- 1 cup dates, pitted and soaked for 1 hour in water, then rough chopped
- 2 cups carrots, shredded
- 1 ½ cups apple, minced
- 1 ½ cups raw cashews or pecans, ground into a fine meal
- ½ tsp cinnamon, freshly ground
- ½ tsp nutmeg, freshly ground
- ½ tsp sea salt

> " I love maple sugar as a natural sweetener for its beautiful maple aromatherapy that brings back my childhood memories of hiking in the woods. It adds beauty and mindfulness to the cooking process, such as when making the Apple Crisp and Sweet Potato Brownie. "

SIMPLE STEPS

1. Gather mise en place.
2. Soak dates.
3. Place all ingredients into mixing bowl and combine gently unit the mixture forms a ball.
4. Press dough into springform pan or bowl.
5. Refrigerate for an hour.
6. Serve with sorbet, fresh fruit, or herbs.

6 Favorite Natural Sweeteners

1. **Dates.** Grow on date palm trees in warm climates, like Arizona. Soak Medjool dates in warm water to make a paste for baking. Dates offer a healthy energy boost. Add to smoothies and use in raw and baked desserts.

2. **Raw local honey.** Buy raw honey at your local farmers' market or directly from local beekeepers. Drizzle on breakfast whole grains and fruit.

3. **Maple syrup and maple sugar.** Sap extracted from maple trees. Darker Grade B contains more antioxidants than Grade A. Maple sugar adds a rich taste and aroma to baked cakes and brownies.

4. **Coconut sugar or coconut palm sugar.** Extracted from the blooms of coconut trees, heated, and evaporated. Caramel color and taste are similar to those of brown sugar. Ideal for baking.

5. **Blackstrap molasses.** Produced during cane sugar processing after sugar crystals are removed. Rich and bittersweet. Works well in baking.

6. **Lucuma.** A tropical fruit native to the highlands of Peru, Chili, and Ecuador. Great when added to smoothies or as a natural sweetener in cookies.

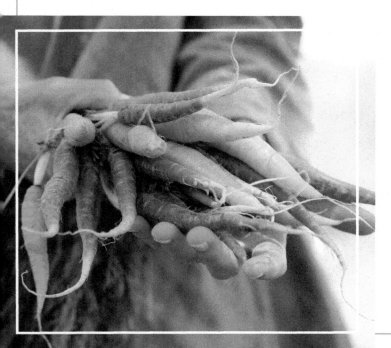

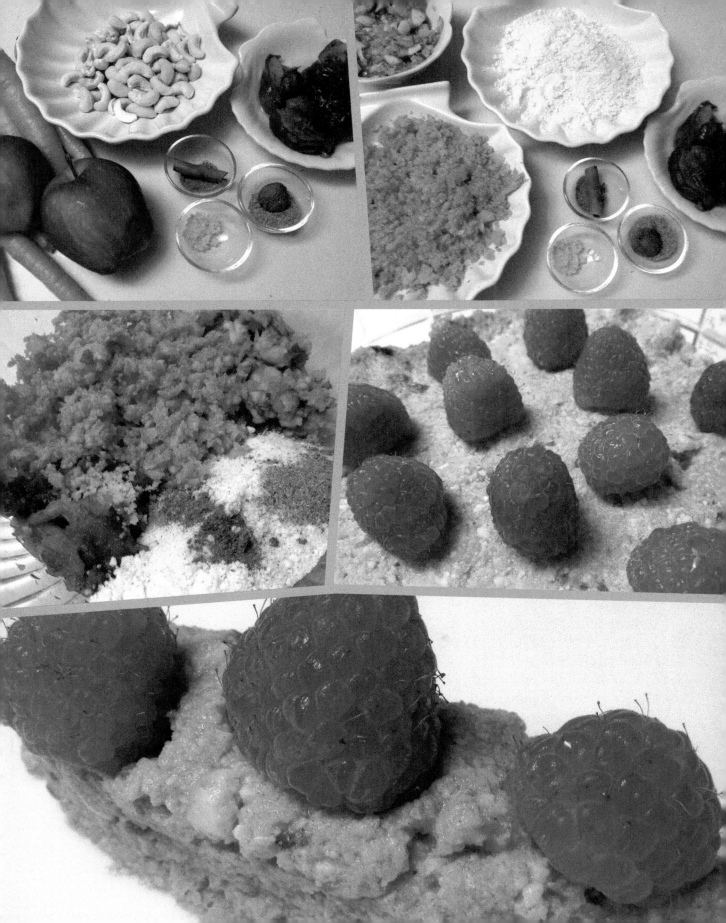

Savory olives and organic sprouted spelt flatbread are excellent snacks and appetizers.

Rosemary Citrus Olives

Olives with fresh rosemary, citrus zest, and garlic are a unique snack, full of natural aromatherapy. Enjoy the mindfulness of zesting citrus and the beauty of different olives, such as Kalamata, and various green and black olives. Try a jar of mixed green olives for a variety of colors and textures in your snack or appetizer.

SIMPLE INGREDIENTS

- ½ cup organic extra virgin olive oil
- 4 garlic cloves, peeled and crushed
- 1 orange, zested
- 1 lemon, zested
- 1 sprig fresh rosemary, torn into ½-inch to 1-inch pieces
- 2 dried bay leaves
- 2 cups olives, with pits

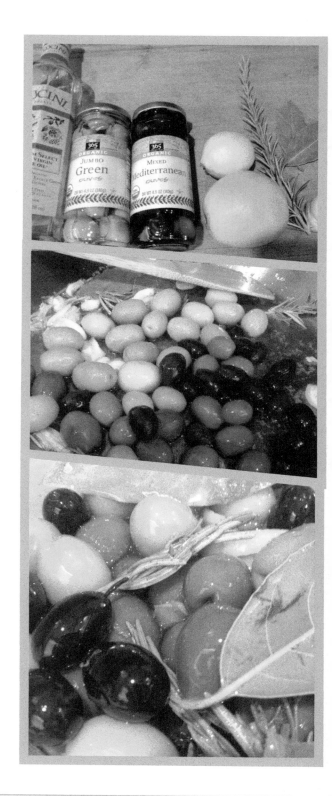

SIMPLE STEPS

1. Gather mise en place.
2. Heat olive oil and garlic in large sauté pan on medium-low heat.
3. Cook for about 3 minutes, until the garlic begins to turn golden.
4. Add the lemon and orange zest, rosemary sprigs, and bay leaves.
5. Stir and let sizzle for about 2 minutes.
6. Add the olives and toss to coat.
7. Transfer to a bowl and let cool.
8. Cover and refrigerate, stirring occasionally.
9. To serve, warm olives and marinate in a pan and reheat over low until warmed, about 2-3 minutes.

Organic Sprouted Spelt Flatbread

A few years ago I discovered that I was sensitive to gluten (the protein in grains like wheat, barley, and rye). By exploring different grain flours, I've found that I'm not sensitive (no hives, no bloating, no headaches) to the Organic Sprouted Spelt Flour by One Degree Organic Foods. Have fun making your own flatbread with this simple recipe.

SIMPLE INGREDIENTS

- ¾ cup hot (not boiling) water
- 1 tbsp dry yeast
- ½ tbsp honey
- 2 tbsp organic olive oil
- 2 cups organic sprouted spelt flour
- ½ tsp sea salt

SIMPLE STEPS

1. Pre-heat oven to 500 degrees F with pizza brick in the oven.
2. Put dry yeast, honey, and olive oil into a cup with hot water.
3. Let it sit for about 10 minutes.
4. Pour sprouted spelt flour and sea salt in a bowl.
5. Add the water with yeast into the flour mixture.
6. Blend with a fork for a few minutes, then knead with your hands for another few minutes. Only knead for about 3-4 minutes total; otherwise, the flatbread will be tough. If the dough is sticky, add more flour. If it's dry, add more water.
7. Coat a large bowl with olive oil. Place dough in bowl, cover with a towel, and rest for about 15 minutes. Any additional water in the dough will soak into the flour.
8. Split the dough in half. Place 2 balls of dough into the bowl coated with olive oil, and cover for about 2 hours (to rise).
9. Again, split the dough into 2 sections and spread it onto a pizza brick using your hands.
10. Bake for 5 minutes, then check for doneness (crispy on outside and soft on inside). Bake for another 3-5 minutes if needed.
11. Enjoy.

❝ This Organic Sprouted Spelt Flatbread has become a staple in my home and when I travel. This year I made the flatbread with 15 pounds of the flour and my family and friends from Florida to Arizona all enjoyed its simplicity. ❞

5 Ways to Enjoy Organic Sprouted Spelt Flatbread

1. Side with Rosemary Citrus Olives
2. Drizzle with olive oil and freshly chopped basil
3. Dip into tomatoes, olive oil, and balsamic vinegar
4. Use as a pizza crust and top with sautéed farmers' market veggies
5. Just plain

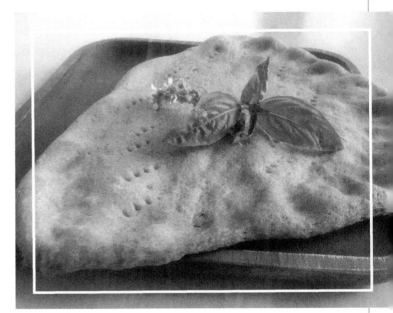

Action : Superfoods, Desserts, and Snacks.

In this section, we've explored several different superfoods, as well as several incredible ways to prepare amazing chocolate desserts, fruit sorbet, and carrot cake, along with some savory snacks and my favorite Organic Sprouted Spelt Flatbread. I invite you to experiment with a chocolate dessert and a savory snack. Have fun creating these gourmet-quality dishes.

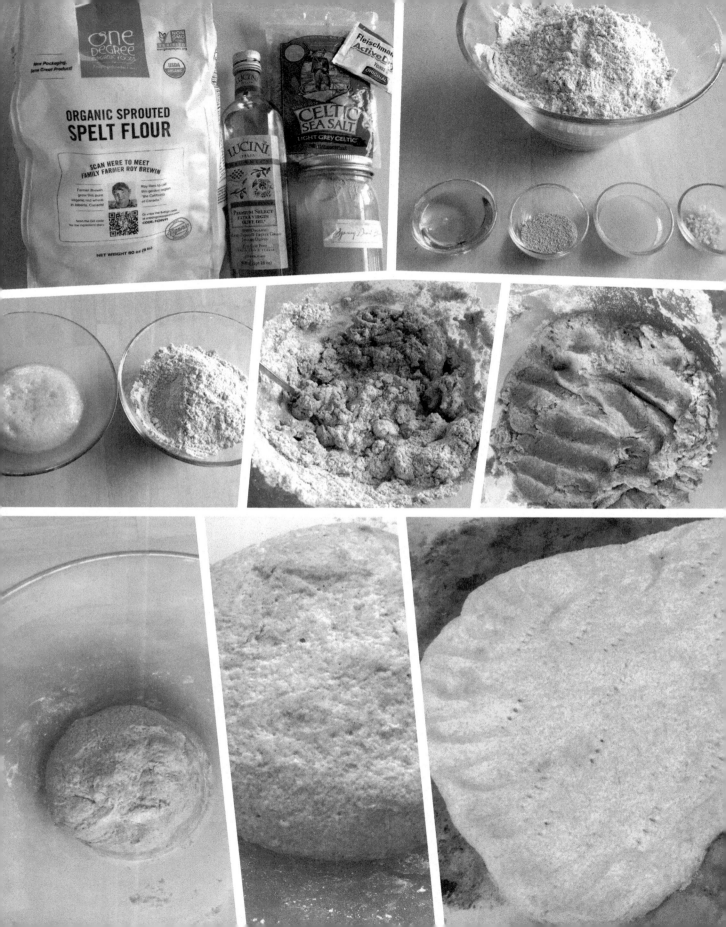

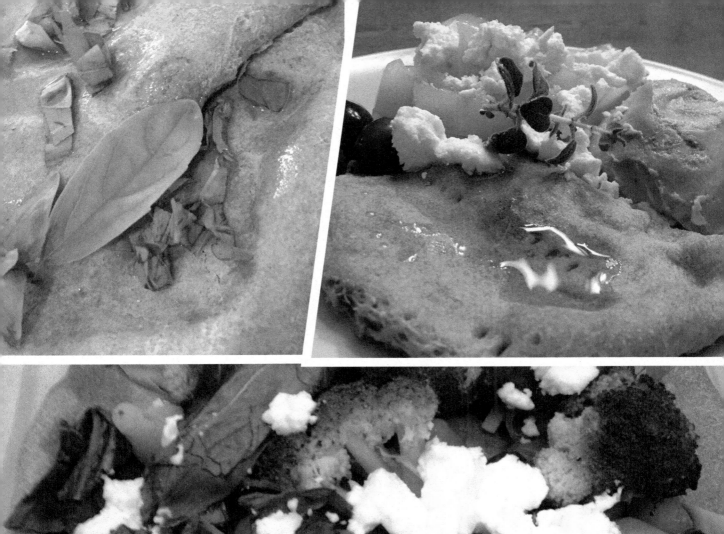
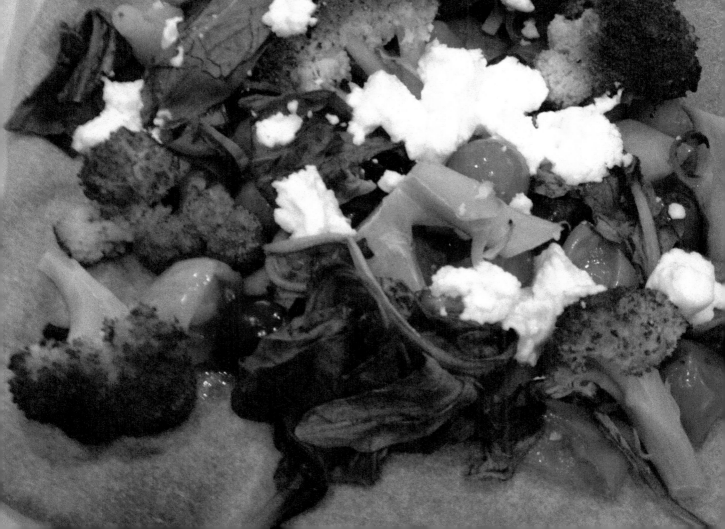

Drink Green Tea, Root Tea and No Recipe Smoothies

Culinary
- Basic tea accessories
- Tips to purchase high-quality tea
- Most popular green teas
- What's the difference: loose leaf tea vs. tea bags
- No recipe smoothies: 5 simple steps to create an intuitive smoothie

Recipes
- 4 simple steps to prepare matcha tea
- 5 simple steps to steep the perfect green tea
- Experience root tea: ginger and turmeric root

Nutrition
- Why we must hydrate
- Signs of dehydration
- How much water to drink
- Top 6 reasons why green tea is good for you
- Why coconut water is great for hydration

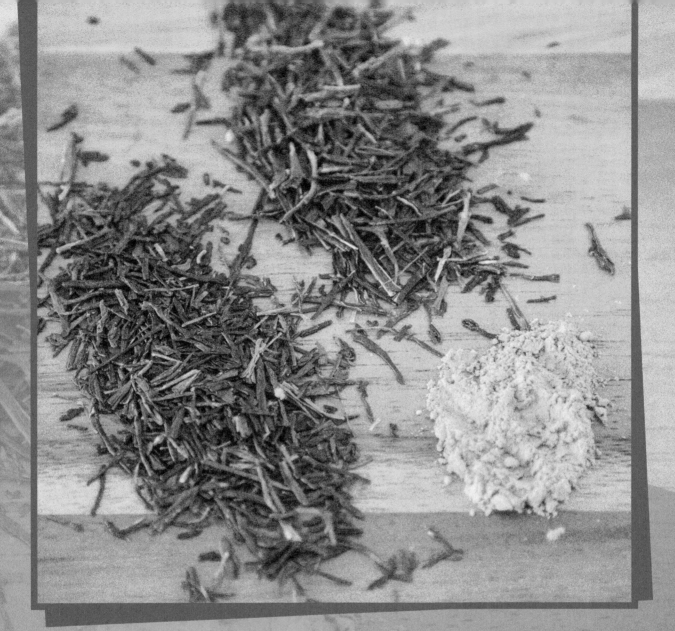

DRINK GREEN TEA, ROOT TEA AND NO RECIPE
SMOOTHIES

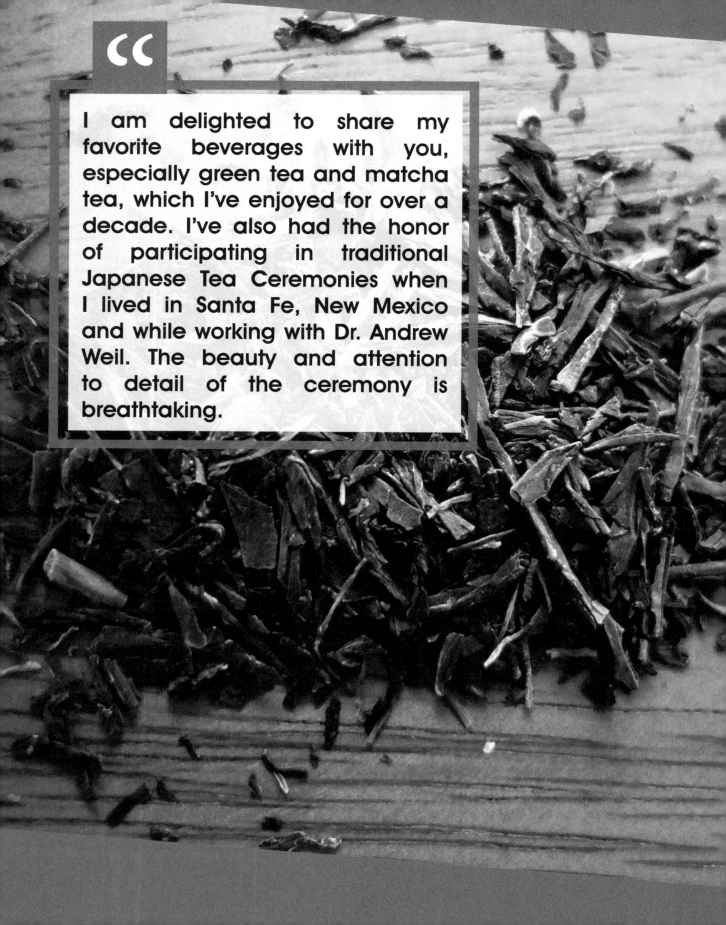

I am delighted to share my favorite beverages with you, especially green tea and matcha tea, which I've enjoyed for over a decade. I've also had the honor of participating in traditional Japanese Tea Ceremonies when I lived in Santa Fe, New Mexico and while working with Dr. Andrew Weil. The beauty and attention to detail of the ceremony is breathtaking.

DRINK GREEN TEA, ROOT TEA AND NO RECIPE SMOOTHIES

Let's drink healthy beverages

Unfortunately so many people drink soft drinks and other beverages full of sugar and other additives. In addition, many people are often dehydrated. In this section, we'll explore why hydration is vital to our health and learn about the top healthy beverages. You'll discover how to prepare and enjoy green tea and the matcha tea ritual, make root tea with fresh ginger and turmeric root, and learn to intuitively make delicious smoothies without recipes.

We will explore:
- Why we must stay hydrated
- Benefits of drinking green tea
- Why ginger and turmeric are good for us
- Benefits of coconut water

You'll learn how to:
- Make a perfect cup of matcha tea
- Steep loose leaf green tea
- Brew ginger root and turmeric root tea
- Mix and match ingredients to create your own intuitive smoothies without using recipes

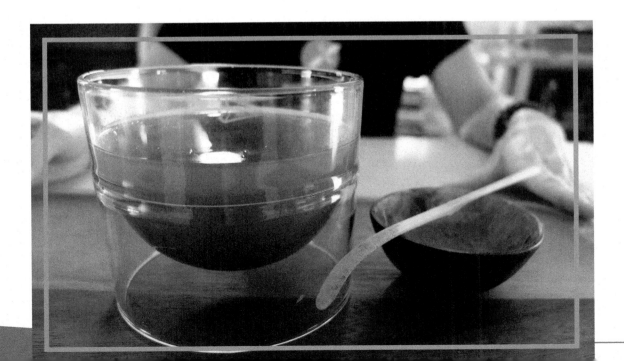

WHY HYDRATE?

Before we explore different ways to hydrate, it's important to understand why hydration is vital to our health.

Our Systems Need Water

Our bodies are 75% water and our brains are 85% water; every system needs water to function properly. Water:

- Carries nutrients to cells.
- Is essential for proper digestion.
- Lubricates joints and is important for all movement.
- Helps excrete waste and toxins from the body.
- Regulates body temperature.

Stay Hydrated for Health

- **Heart:** Dehydration lowers the blood volume, requiring our heart to work harder to provide enough oxygen to cells.
- **Brain:** Staying hydrated keeps the memory sharp and the mood stable. Even slight dehydration reduces our ability to recall new information.
- **Exercise:** Dehydration makes exercise and even walking more difficult, and reduces the amount of aerobic exercise we can do.

Water Loss Can Negatively Impact Your Body

As little as a 0.5% reduction in bodyweight due to water loss can strain our hearts, and as little as a 1% reduction can reduce performance during exercise. Several studies have reported that being dehydrated, especially when it's hot, reduces the amount of aerobic exercise you can do; people who were just slightly dehydrated were typically able to run only 75% as hard as usual.

Effect of Water Loss on Your Health

Percent Reduction in Bodyweight Due to Water Loss

0.5%	Increased strain on heart
1%	Reduced aerobic activity
3%	Reduced muscular endurance
4%	Reduced muscle strength, reduced motor skills, heat cramps
5%	Heat exhaustion, cramping, fatigue, reduced mental capacity
6%	Physical exhaustion, cramping, fatigue, reduced mental clarity
10-20%	Death

How Much Water Do You Need to Drink?

It depends on you. The amount of water you need to drink depends on your size, age, level of physical activity, and geographical location. Do you exercise often? Do you live in a warm, dry climate? Are you older? You should drink more water if you reside in a hot, dry climate like Arizona or if you work out often. If you are over 65 with medical conditions, it's important to consult your healthcare provider about proper fluid intake, as too much water may be as dangerous as too little.

Ideal Daily Water Intake

To determine how much water you should be drinking:

- Take your weight in pounds and divide it by 2 to get the number of ounces you should drink daily. As an example, if you weigh 150 pounds, you should drink about 75 ounces of water every day. That's a little more than a half-gallon of water a day, or 10 8-ounce cups.
- Add extra ounces if you exercise often or live in a hot, dry climate.

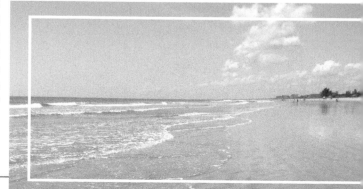

Get Clear on Dehydration

Since hydration is important, it's valuable to understand the signs of dehydration, from mild to severe.

Mild Dehydration

If it occurs frequently, mild dehydration may increase the risk of health problems such as heartburn, constipation, kidney stones, and even kidney failure. Mild dehydration happens when we lose 3-5% of bodyweight through the loss of fluids (usually sweat, vomit, or diarrhea). When we're already low on fluids, and we exercise or do physical labor in a hot environment, we can become dehydrated in a few hours.

Fortunately, dehydration triggers significant thirst, so if you feel thirsty, listen to your body and take frequent sips of water. Don't consume too much water too quickly, especially if you're suffering from nausea or diarrhea – it's likely to make things worse. The first signs of mild dehydration are a headache and flushed red face.

Signs of Mild Dehydration

- Thirst
- Headache
- Flushed, red face
- Dizziness or lightheadedness
- Tiredness with no energy
- Dry skin
- Dry mouth
- Chills
- Muscle weakness
- Dark-colored urine
- Reduced urine output

Severe Dehydration

Severe dehydration can cause our bodies to shut down and go into shock. Make sure you know the early warning signs of dehydration so that you can take action and protect your health.

Signs of Severe Dehydration

- Extreme thirst
- Little or no urine
- Lack of sweating
- Low blood pressure
- Rapid heartbeat
- Fever
- Irritability and confusion
- Very dry mouth, skin, and mucous membranes
- Shriveled and dry skin that lacks elasticity and doesn't "bounce back" when pinched
- Sunken eyes
- Delirium or unconsciousness in most serious cases

Quick Dehydration Check

Check if you're dehydrated by answering these three simple questions and commit to being serious about hydration.

1. Are you thirsty?
2. Is your morning urine dark yellow, like apple juice?
3. Is your body weight more than a few pounds (1%) lower than it was yesterday morning?

If you answer YES to one question, you might be dehydrated. If you answer YES to two questions, you are likely dehydrated. If you answer YES to all three questions, you are very likely dehydrated.

> " Hydration is so important to health and life. Be sure to hydrate all day, every day. "

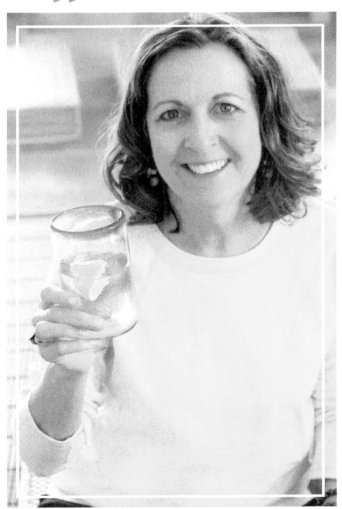

GET READY TO ENJOY GREEN TEA

I began drinking green tea over a decade ago in 2004 when I started working in marketing and licensing with best-selling author and integrative medicine pioneer, Dr. Andrew Weil, who has been a long-time advocate of drinking green tea.

My green tea experience grew from bitter to mindful. When I first started drinking loose green tea, I found it to be very bitter tasting, but I kept experimenting with different teas and even attended The World Tea Expo for a few years. Importantly, I learned the proper way to brew green tea for an enjoyable, smooth taste. Today I love the smooth, grassy taste, along with the mindful experience of brewing and enjoying tea.

Start with High-quality Tea

To really enjoy tea, be prepared with high-quality tea and the right tea accessories. Purchase a few different high-quality loose green teas. Start with 1-2 ounces of green teas such as Sencha and Gyokuro.

Top 6 Reasons Why Green Tea is Good for You

1. The antioxidant ECGC, in green tea, is an anti-inflammatory.
2. Research has found that green tea benefits heart health and brain health, and helps prevent cancer.
3. It is full of catechins and polyphenols, which help the brain relax and stimulate dopamine levels.
4. Theanine in green tea helps improve mood and provides a sense of relaxation.
5. Green tea has less caffeine than coffee.
6. It tastes delicious, so enjoy a few cups every day.

3 Popular Green Teas

Matcha: Tea of the Japanese tea ceremony
- High quality Japanese green tea is covered before picking to accentuate its vibrant green color and to increase amino acids, as well as vitamins A and C.
- The tea leaves are stone-ground, so we actually eat tea leaves when we drink matcha tea and receive the full benefits of green tea.
- Intense grassy, green taste.

Gyokuro: High-quality Japanese tea
- The tea bushes are covered for two weeks prior to harvesting with nets or trellises to reduce the amount of sunlight the plants receive.
- The emerald leaf takes on a lustrous, splinter-like appearance.
- Deep, intense, rich green color and grassy, fresh taste.

Sencha: Most popular Japanese tea
- An excellent starting point for those just beginning to explore green tea.
- The splintered green leaf delivers a vegetal, yellow-green cup.
- In Japan, Sencha is served hot in the cooler months and usually chilled in the summer months.

" Mindfully experiment with a few green teas: matcha, gyokuro, and sencha. "

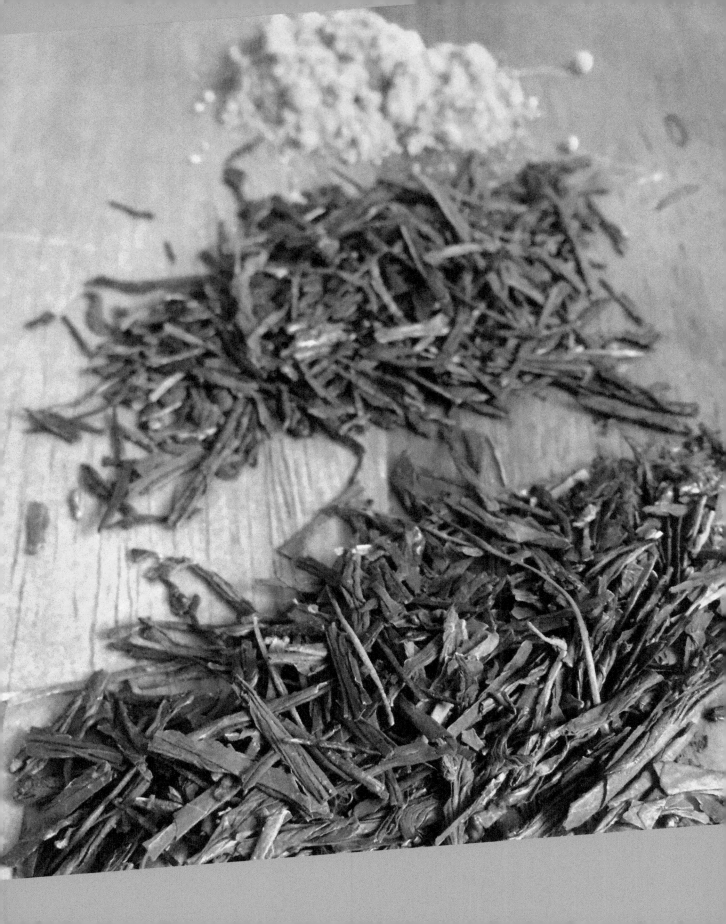

GET READY WITH 8 BASIC TEA ACCESSORIES

With these tea essentials, you will enjoy the mindful experience of brewing and drinking tea.

1. **Tea kettle.** Enamel or stainless steel tea kettle to heat water on the stove.
2. **Teapot.** Pot to brew tea. I love the Chantal teapot with tea strainer. I make green tea in the pot and add water as needed to enjoy all day.
3. **Tea cup.** A few of your favorite glass cups to enjoy drinking tea.
4. **Tea canisters.** Tea tins to keep high-quality loose leaf tea out of the light.
5. **Tea balls.** Stainless steel balls to brew loose tea, such as these antique tea balls that were my grandmother's.
6. **Matcha tea bowl.** Special bowl to prepare matcha tea, such as our Super Bowl XLII matcha tea bowl.
7. **Bamboo whisk.** Japanese tea ceremony Chasen whisk to prepare matcha tea.
8. **Bamboo spoon.** Bamboo scoop to dish out matcha tea powder.

Drink Green, Like the Japanese

In Japanese populations, green tea consumption has been linked to longer life, especially among people drinking five cups or more daily. Western populations consume relatively little green tea.

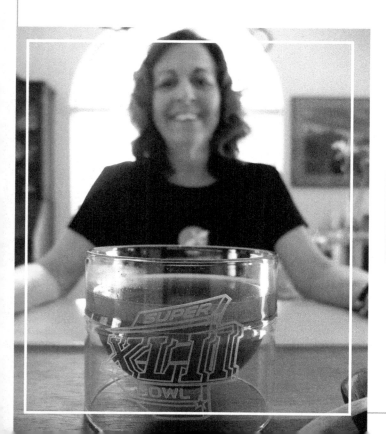

What's the Difference: Loose Leaf Tea vs. Tea Bags

Loose Leaf Tea

- Loose leaf tea is actual tea leaves, which may be a specialty tea from a single region of the world.
- Flavor is extracted from whole leaves that expand in warm water.
- Steep the same leaves multiple times for several cups of tea.

Tea Bags

- Often contain low-grade tea dust and fannings from broken tea leaves, which lose their essential oils and aroma.
- When steeped, broken tea leaves release more tannins than whole leaf teas, resulting in a bitter, astringent flavor.
- Generally, tea bags can be used for only one cup of tea.

> " Enjoying matcha and green tea is a beautiful, mindful daily ritual in my life. I invite you to add the experience of enjoying green tea to your life. "

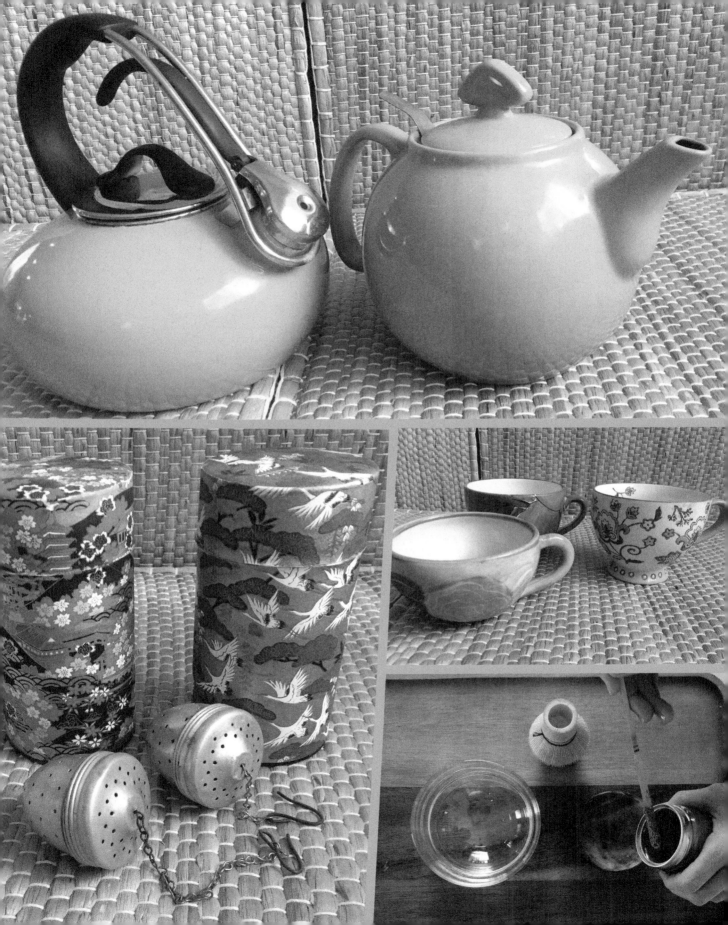

EXPERIENCE GREEN TEA

5 Simple Steps to Steep the Perfect Green Tea

Take the time to try a Japanese green loose tea, such as the high-quality Gyokuro or Sencha, the most popular Japanese tea. The key is to brew your tea properly so that it is not bitter tasting.

1. Put 1 teaspoon of loose tea leaves in a tea ball or 2-3 teaspoons in the teapot strainer.
2. Bring a few cups of water to almost a boil.
3. Pour water over the tea leaves.
4. Cover the pot or cup and steep for 2-3 minutes.
5. Continue steeping the tea leaves with warm water and enjoy your green tea throughout the day.

Do not burn green tea leaves

Green tea leaves are very delicate because they are minimally processed. When steeping green tea, use very warm (not boiling) water so that you do not burn the fragile tea leaves. Many people burn the leaves when they make green tea and then don't care for the bitterness of it.

4 Simple Steps to Prepare Matcha Tea

1. Place ¼ tsp matcha in matcha bowl.
2. Add nearly boiled water.
3. Whisk with a bamboo whisk.
4. Enjoy the ritual and ceremony.

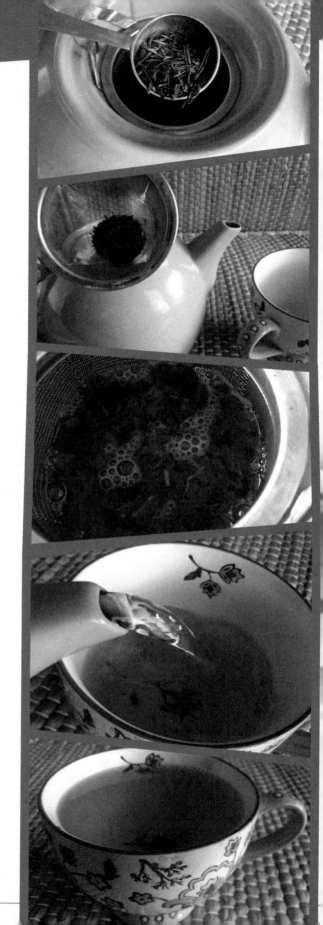

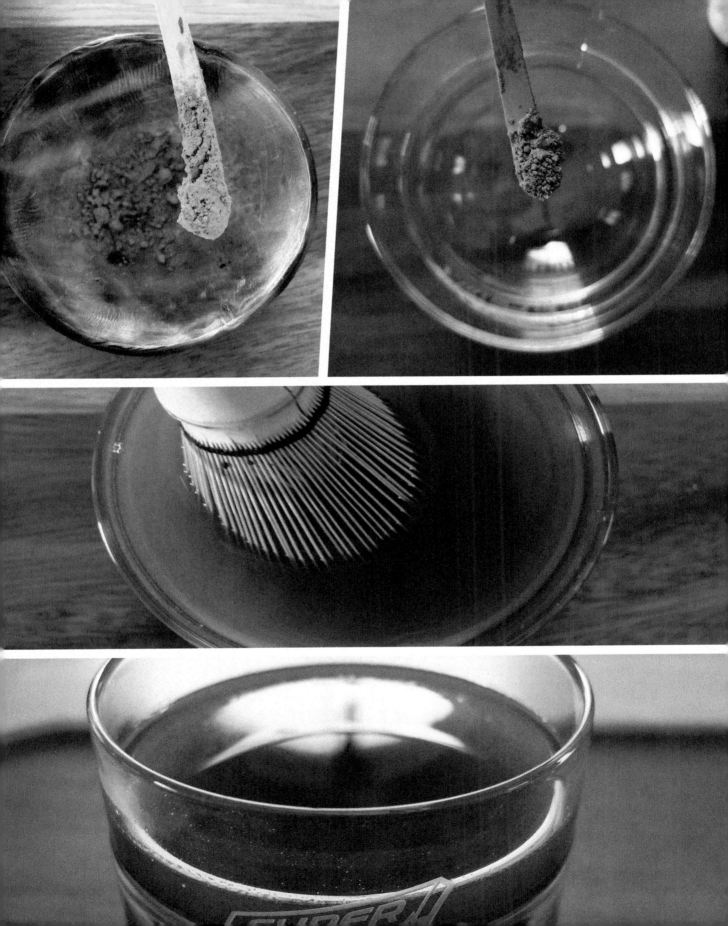

EXPERIENCE ROOT TEA

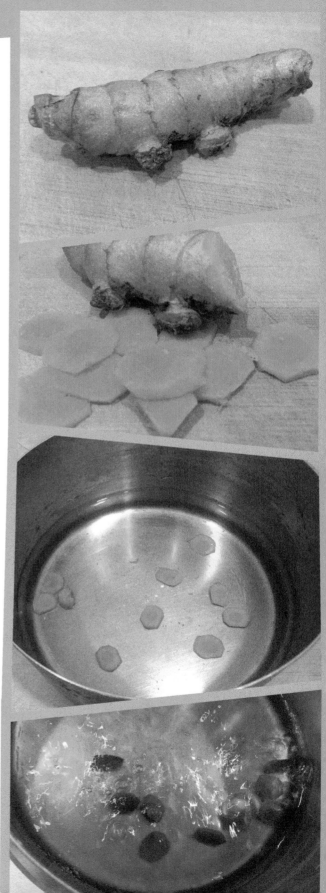

Ginger and turmeric herbs are tropical plants whose roots are used medicinally and as beverages. Ginger and turmeric tea have been popular in Asia for centuries. Ginger tea is very common in China. Turmeric tea is an everyday drink in Okinawa, Japan, home to the world's highest known concentration of centenarians.

Ginger Root

- Natural anti-inflammatory
- Reduces nausea and helps digestion
- Beneficial for colds and the flu

Turmeric Root

- Used medicinally in India and China for centuries
- Contains curcumin, an anti-inflammatory known to alleviate arthritis and reduce muscle pain and joint inflammation
- Thermogenic properties that increase metabolism and fat burning, which aid in the increasing of energy and weight loss

6 Steps to Make Root Tea

1. Slice ginger or turmeric root into thin slices without skin.
2. Place into a small pot of water.
3. Add black pepper to turmeric to enhance its healing properties.
4. Bring water to boil.
5. Simmer for 10-15 minutes.
6. If desired, add honey for sweetness.

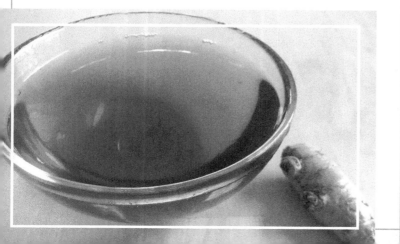

Smoothies

Smoothies are a perfect way to eat a variety of organic fruit and veggies and a simple morning meal or afternoon snack. Because we drink all of the nutrients and fiber in smoothies, they're nutritious and slow the digestive process. Make your own smoothies with your intuition using these steps. Have fun mixing and matching the ingredients in your smoothies based on what's available in season and your own cravings.

No-Recipe Smoothies: 5 Simple Steps to Create an Intuitive Smoothie

1. Pour 1 cup of non-dairy liquid into a high-speed blender.
   - Coconut water
   - Homemade nut milk (coconut water with almonds or soaked cashews)
   - Homemade seed milk (coconut water with hemp seeds or sunflower seeds)
   - 1 date for sweetness
   - 1 teaspoon of vanilla extract for smoothness

2. Add a thickening ingredient to liquid and blend.
   - Avocado
   - Bananas, frozen or fresh
   - Chia seeds; use 1 tablespoon of seeds and 3 tablespoons of liquid, pre-soaked for 10 minutes

3. Add about ¼ cup fruit, fresh or frozen.
   - Apple, sliced
   - Cherries
   - Berries: blueberries, raspberries, strawberries

4. Add about ¼ cup vegetables.
   - Carrots
   - Celery
   - Cucumber
   - Kale
   - Spinach

5. Add other extras.
   - Flaxseeds
   - Fresh basil or mint
   - Ginger or turmeric root
   - Goji berries
   - Raw cacao powder

Get to Know Coconut Water

Coconut water is the juice in the interior or endosperm of young coconuts. It is clear, sweet, sterile, and about 95% water.

Why Coconut Water is Great for Hydration

- High in the electrolyte potassium. Eleven ounces of coconut water contains 610 mg of potassium. For perspective, the adult daily requirement for potassium is 4,700 mg.
  - Aids in our body's water absorption.
  - Low potassium is associated with a risk of high blood pressure, heart disease, stroke, arthritis, cancer, digestive disorders, and infertility.
- Full of water
  - Muscles: Helps contraction and relaxation of muscles
  - Heart: Helps balance blood pressure

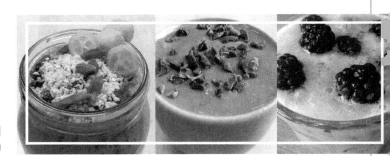

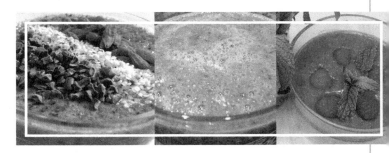

Action : Green Tea, Root Tea, and Smoothies

In this section, we've explored several healthy beverages and learned how to prepare them. If you're new to green tea and matcha, I invite you to try green tea and enjoy the mindful experience of preparing it. If you are new to root tea, brew a pot of ginger or turmeric root tea and notice how you feel when drinking it. Finally, enjoy making your own intuitively created smoothies without recipes. Experiment with different combinations of liquids, nuts, seeds, fruits, and vegetables. Enjoy!

Thank You

Creative Team
- Kostis Pavlou, Book Cover
- Suzena Sengupta: Book Interior
- Melissa Corter: Brand and Book Photography
- Henry Dupuis: Food Photography

Organizations and Clients
- Sports
- Youth
- Community
- Wellness
- Holistic

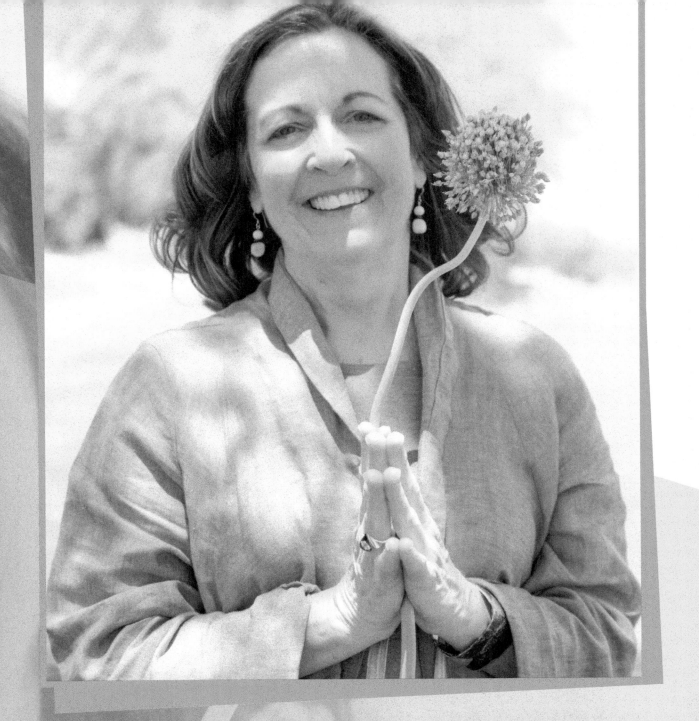

THANK YOU

THANK YOU CREATIVE TEAM

Thanks so much to my international creative team who have worked alongside me for months to bring my passions and the vision of my book to life in such a beautiful way. I have loved the teamwork and all the dedication and commitment from each of you. Thanks so much!

Kostis Pavlou: Book Cover

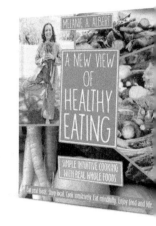

Thanks so much to Kostis Pavlou in Greece, who is the designer of the cover of *A New View of Healthy Eating*. Thanks Kostis for your fresh, fun, energizing design that provided the foundation for the look and feel of the book. From the moment that I saw your design my intuition told me that this was the look for the book. Thank you for your amanzing creativity and it was a joy working with you.

Kostis Pavlou is one of the lucky people blessed enough to remember almost their every dream. One of his favorite is when he saw himself being recreated one pixel at a time by Storm Thogerson and obtain weird limbs and eyes by Salvador Dali's brush. His surrealistic perception of things as well as his repugnance for anything realistic around him, pushed him towards the arts. He has come a long way since being a graphic artist in the small town of Katerini, transforming into a traveller of digital collage and a huntsman of the implausible: a door on the surface of the sea, a car in the clouds and an elephant in his desk drawer.

Melissa Corter: Brand and Book Photography

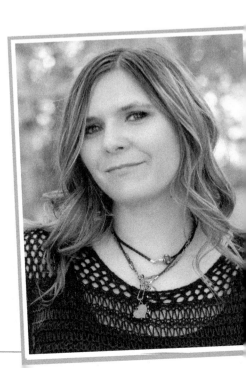

Thanks so much to my friend Melissa Corter from Sedona, Arizona, who beautifully captured the look and feel of my brand and book through her camera with her calm, loving way of taking photos. Our branding and lifestyle photoshoot was a fun collaboration. I love the photos taken at your retreat in Sedona and our shoot in one of my favorite places at my home at the Legacy Golf Resort.

Melissa is a spiritual teacher, author, and soul artist. She has a gift of capturing the essence of her clients, while providing a safe space, and unconditional love to help them release their fears of "being seen".

Suzena Samuel: Book Interior

Special thanks to Suzena in New Delhi India, who is the incredible designer of the interior of the book. Suzena and I spent many weeks working together as she page-by-page brought my passions and the vision of my book to life so beautifully. I appreciate your creativity, passion for design, attention to detail, and always positive outlook. I love the design from my heart and it has been so much fun working together on the book.

The dream to make a living out of books and wanting alternatively to write stories and illustrating them led her to her love for beautiful book covers and layouts. She would spend hours sketching and writing stories as a child. The desire to learn and create, had her pursue design diploma in fine arts, illustration and graphics while graduating in advertising. She works as an Art Editor and freelancer, designing books and their covers.

Painting and Reading are her two great loves. She is also mommy to her two year old son 'Shaurya' and two wonderful dogs 'Cherry and Tia'. It is often loud, chaotic and full of giggles and hugs and licks at her home. And that is her secret to creativity and happy energy that comes across in her designs.

Henry Dupuis: Food Photography

Thanks to artist Henry Dupuis, who has followed his dreams and is living in Australia, for the fun food photo shoot at the farmers' market and up-close food photography in my home. You really have an eye for detail and I appreciate your contribution to my book.

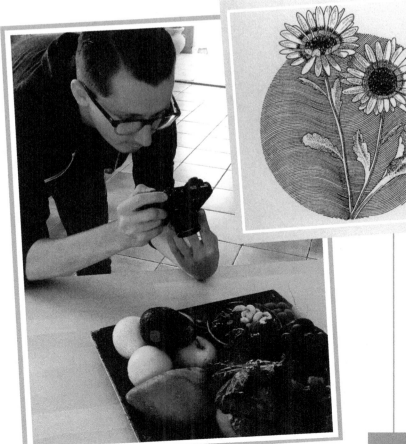

Photo credits
Back Cover: Roots
Pages: 12 (Melanie), 27, 32 (salad),45 (tomatoes, peppers), 65, 66, 83, 84, 85,103,105,139,141,178, 179,184,185 (matcha accessories),187

THANKS PARTNERS AND CLIENTS

Thanks to all the organizations and individuals who have believed in me and supported my passions to enjoy food and enhance health through hands-on interactive food and lifestyle experiences. I appreciate you!

Thank You NFL Super Bowl Events and Former NFL Players

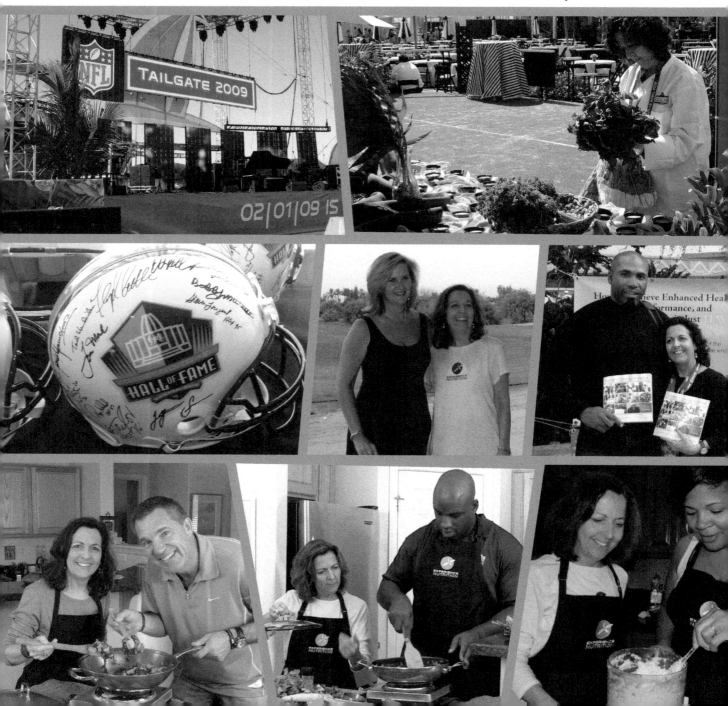

Thank You NFL Alumni Association

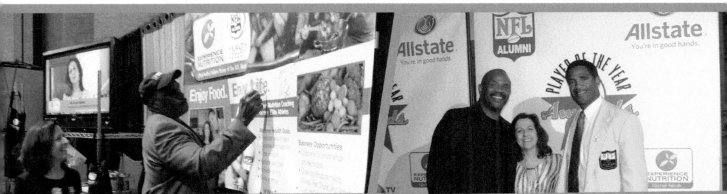

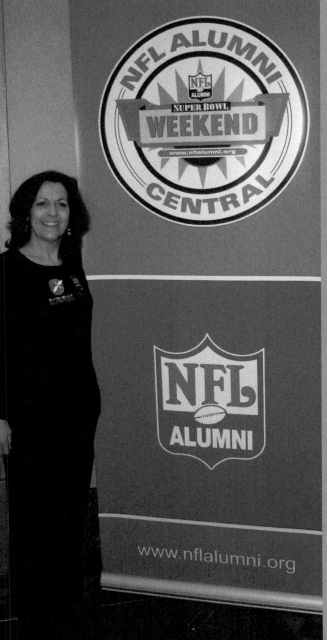

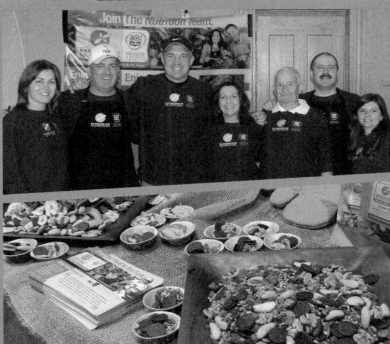

**SPORTS: NFL SUPER BOWL EVENTS AND FORMER NFL PLAYERS
LEFT**
- NFL Super Bowl VIP Tailgate
- NFL Hall of Fame Players Classic
- NFL Hall of Fame Players Classic, Megan Holland
- Super Bowl Champion, Seth Joyner
- Former NFL Quarterback, Dave Krieg
- Former NFL Player, John Bronson
- NFL Wife, Ericka Lassister

**SPORTS: 2011 OFFICIAL HEALTH & WELLNESS PARTNER,
NFL ALUMNI ASSOCIATION
RIGHT**
- Player Networking Event, with former NFL player,
  Charlie Davis
- Player of the Year Awards, with Reggie Haynes
  and Hall of Fame Mike Haynes
- NFL Alumni Central, Super Bowl XLV
- Super Bowl XLIV Week: Experience Nutrition Team
- Experience Nutrition Trail Mix

Thank You Youth Organizations

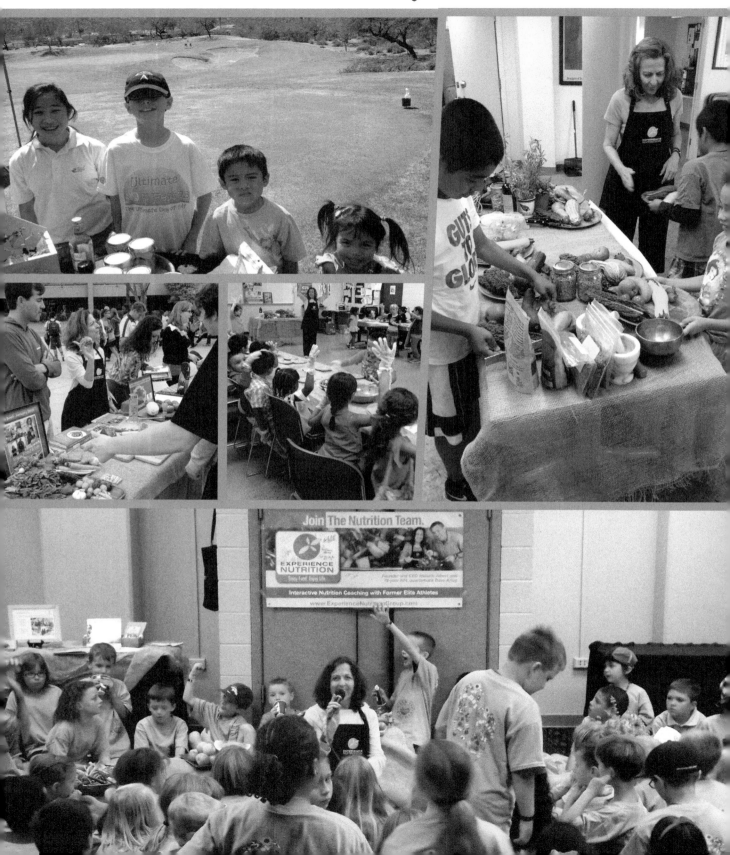

Thank You Wellness

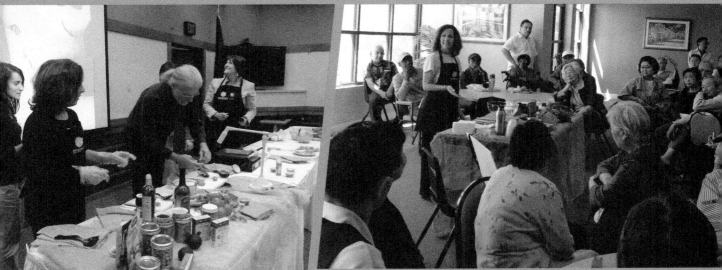

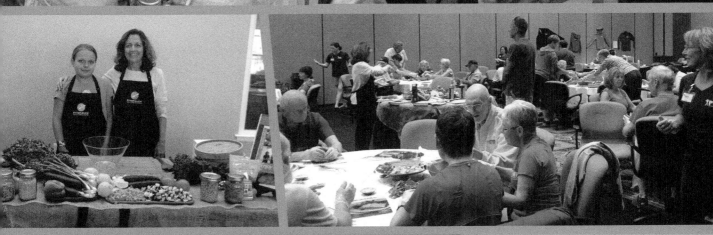

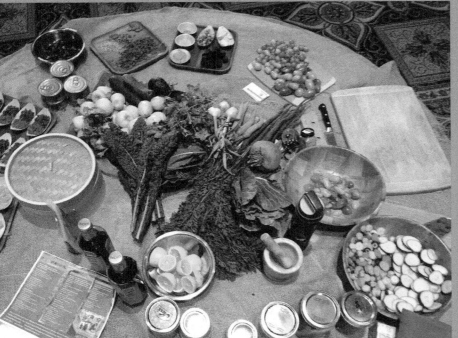

YOUTH ORGANIZATIONS
LEFT
- The First Tee of Phoenix
- Future for Kids
- Desert Vista High School
- Phoenix Youth Sports Day
- Phoenix Suns/
  Phoenix Mercury Kids Camp

WELLNESS
RIGHT
- Marquette General
  Hospital Health Conference
- Gregory's Fresh Market Seniors,
  with "Meredith Albert"
- Parkinson's Wellness Recovery

Thank You Phoenix Community

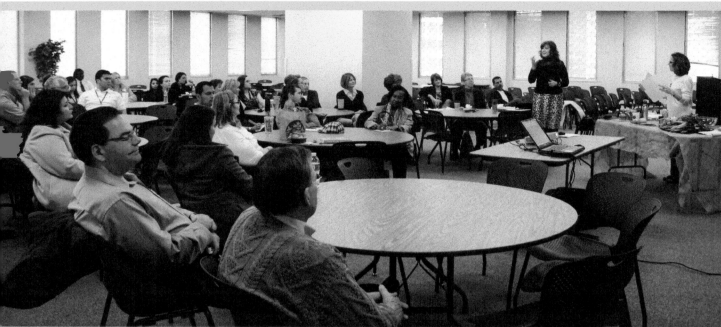

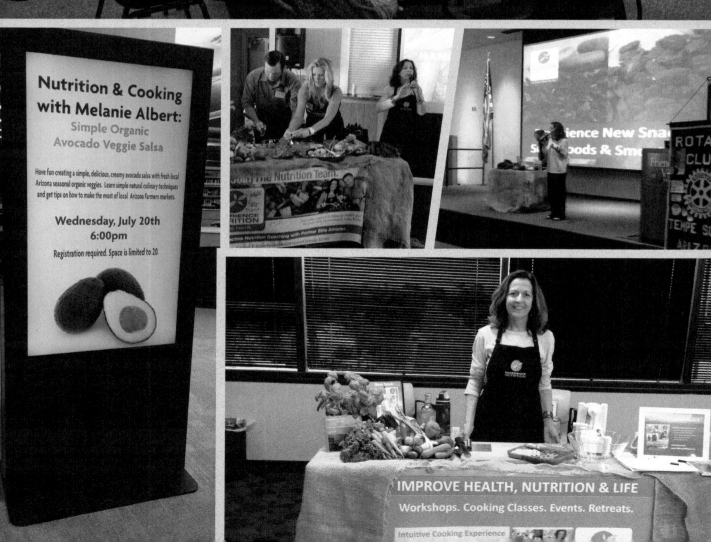

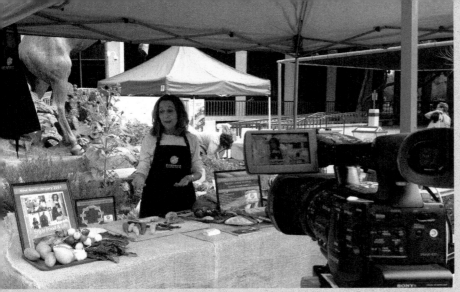

COMMUNITY

LEFT
- City of Phoenix
- Maricopa Library District
- Thrive Health Initiative
- Rotary Club, Tempe, AZ
- Arizona Bar Association

RIGHT
- Earth Day Phoenix
- Maya's Farm
- Phoenix Public Market
- Private Cooking Class, with Tanya Roberts, Audrey Holton Johnson, India Lee Benedetto
- Valley Permaculture Alliance

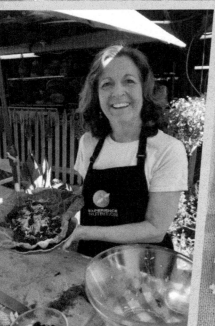
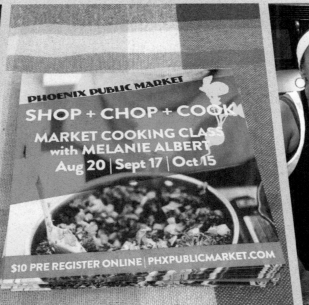
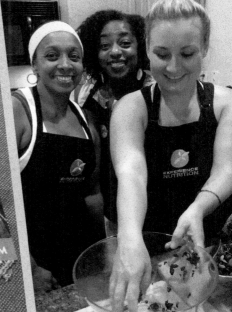

PHOENIX PUBLIC MARKET

SHOP + CHOP + COOK

MARKET COOKING CLASS
with MELANIE ALBERT
Aug 20 | Sept 17 | Oct 15

$10 PRE REGISTER ONLINE | PHXPUBLICMARKET.COM

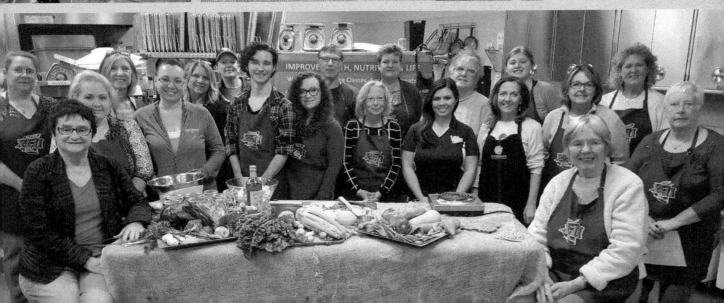

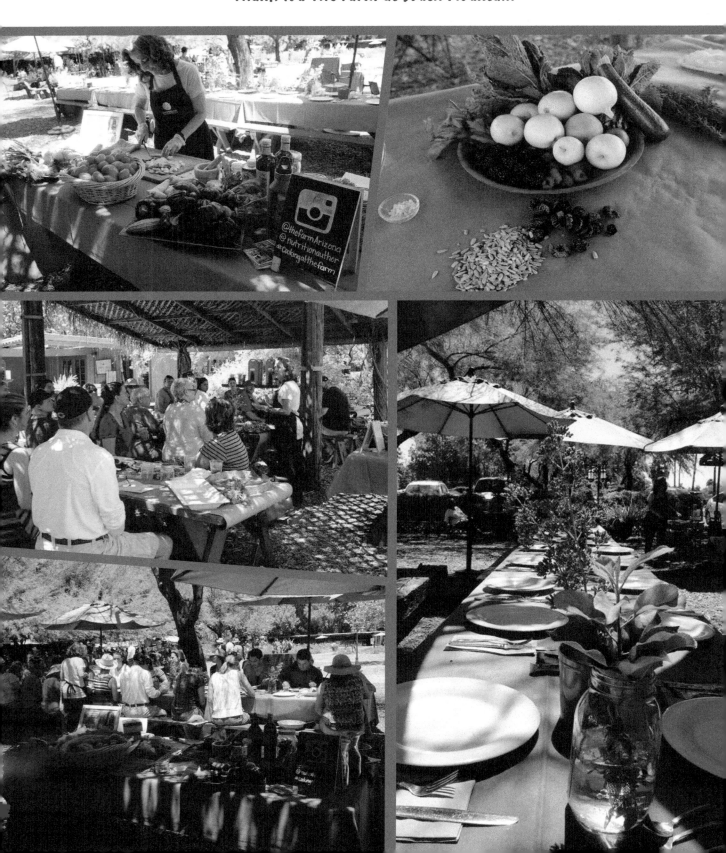

Thank You Holistic Community

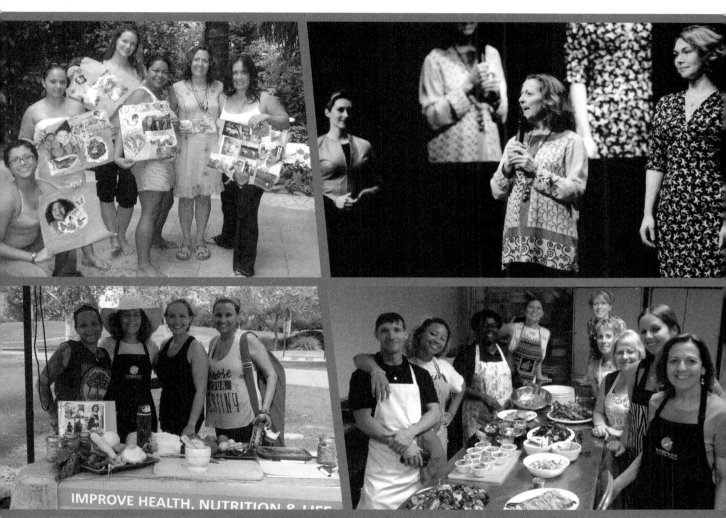

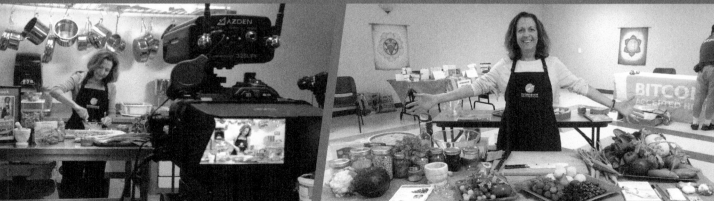

FARM AT SOUTH MOUNTAIN
T

The Farm at South Mountain

HOLISTIC COMMUNITY
RIGHT
- Harmony Hotel, Nosara, Costa Rica
- Institute for Integrative Nutrition
- Yoga Rocks the Park, Phoenix, AZ
- Southwest Institute of Healing Arts

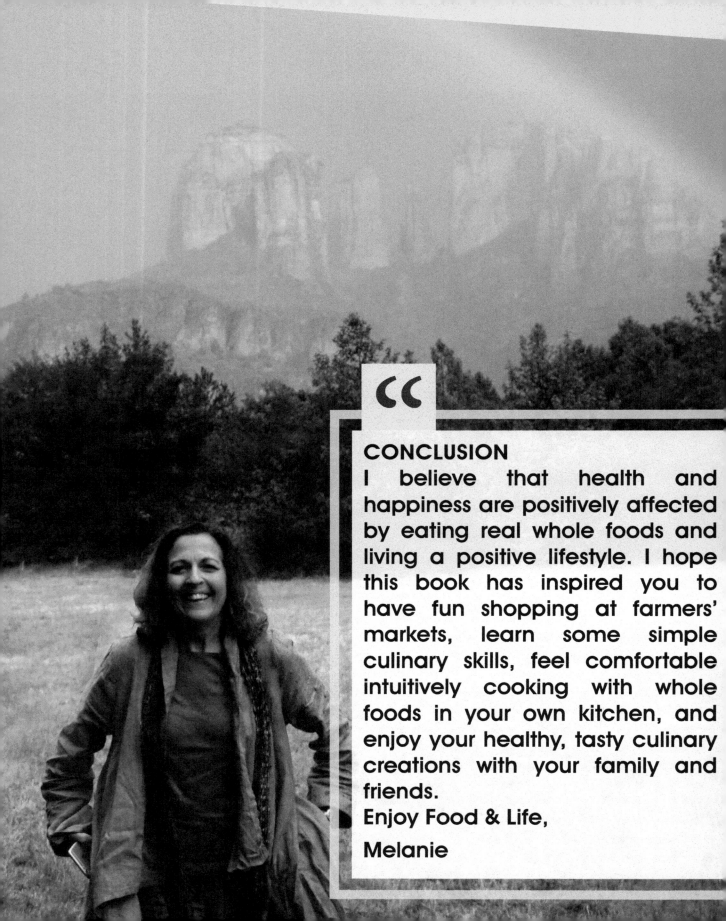

"

CONCLUSION
I believe that health and happiness are positively affected by eating real whole foods and living a positive lifestyle. I hope this book has inspired you to have fun shopping at farmers' markets, learn some simple culinary skills, feel comfortable intuitively cooking with whole foods in your own kitchen, and enjoy your healthy, tasty culinary creations with your family and friends.

Enjoy Food & Life,

Melanie

About the Author

Melanie A. Albert, intuitive cooking expert, author, and speaker, is Founder and CEO of Experience Nutrition Group, LLC, in Phoenix, Arizona. Melanie has been active in wellness, integrative medicine, and nutrition for over 15 years. She is a 2007 graduate of the Institute for Integrative Nutrition in New York City, 2001 Integrative Medicine Fellow and 2003 Intuition Fellow of the Kaiser Institute, former marketing consultant for Weil Lifestyle, LLC / Andrew Weil, MD, current Holistic Nutrition instructor of Whole Foods Cooking and Conscious Eating at the private college Southwest Institute of Healing Arts, in Tempe, Arizona, and 200-hour Registered Yoga Teacher. She received culinary training with the Rouxbe Cooking School Plant-Based Professional Cooking Certification.

Over the last nine years, Melanie has guided thousands of people – former NFL players, MDs, holistic practitioners, office professionals, yoga students, seniors, and kids – through the process of intuitively preparing simple, delicious whole food creations, as well as enjoying food and life. You can always find Melanie shopping at farmers' markets, experimenting in the kitchen, or practicing yoga.

EXPERIENCE NUTRITION improves the lives, health, and nutrition of the holistic and sports communities, organizations, and kids so that they can enjoy healthy food and healthier lives through interactive nutrition education with cooking experiences.

Interested in having Melanie A. Albert speak at your next event?

Melanie has been speaking to groups and organizations for over a decade. She is an expert in intuitive cooking and nutrition and has spoken to thousands of people in Arizona and across the US.

Author of *A New View of Healthy Eating*, Melanie believes that healthy eating begins with the food we choose to eat and extends to our shopping cooking, and eating experiences. The key philosophies are:

- Eat real whole foods.
- Shop local and in season.
- Enjoy intuitive shopping.
- Cook with intuition.
- Eat mindfully.
- Enjoy food and life.

Clients & Partners

Melanie has served as a speaker, workshop, cooking classes, and retreat leader for many organizations including the City of Phoenix, Maricopa Library District, NFL Alumni Association, NFL Hall of Fame Players Classic, The First Tee of Phoenix, Future for Kids, Phoenix Suns/Phoenix Mercury Kids Camp, Phoenix Youth Sports Day, Gregory's Fresh Market, Marquette General Hospital, Parkinson's Wellness Recovery, Sedona Women's Retreat, Flores Wealth Management, Whole Foods Market, Chandler, AZ, Earth Day Phoenix, Food Day Phoenix, The Farm at South Mountain, Valley Permaculture Alliance, Phoenix Pubic Market, Harmony Hotel in Nosara, Costa Rica, Spirt of Yoga, and the Southwest Institute of Healing Arts.

Speaking Topics

Melanie's workshops and cooking classes are fun, interactive and always delicious. In the workshops enjoy interactive cooking experiences, simple culinary techniques, nutrition tips, and mindfully enjoy the organic whole food creations.

Speaking topics, with intuitive cooking class or demo include:

- A New View of Healthy Eating
- Intuitive Cooking with the Season
- Unique Simple Ways to Enjoy Veggies
- Avocado Veggie Salsa
- Organic Raw Kale Salad
- Roots & Greens Stir-fry
- Raw Salads, Cold Soup & Hummus
- Healthy Vegan Desserts
- Hydration & Smoothies

For more information, or to hire Melanie for your next event, call 602.615.2486 or e-mail Mel@MelanieAlbert.com

Visit Melanie online at:

www.facebook.com/NewViewHealthyEating

@nutritionauthor.com

www.EXPNutrition.com